Microbiology

Clinical Microbiology Made Easy

An Introduction and Concise Learning Guide to Master the Fundamentals

Joshua Larsen, MD

Maria Evans, MD

Contents

Section 1: Introduction to Microbiology

Life on earth began with microorganisms, also called microbes or microscopic organisms. Microorganisms are, quite literally, everywhere. The human body itself contains ten times as many microorganisms as it does human cells. Although not immediately obvious, the impact of microorganisms on our lives is enormous. Microorganisms, which can be both useful and harmful, are despite their primarily Gram-negative connotation, central to our health and the health of our ecosystem.

Microbiology is the study of microorganisms and it includes:

• **Morphology:** The study of the form and shape of living cells or organisms, and the relationships between their structures.

• **Metabolism:** The processes that occur within a living cell or organism necessary to maintain life, i.e. how organisms obtain energy from their environment in the form of substances, which are broken down to yield energy and synthesize other substances. Metabolism is studied using biochemistry.

• **Growth:** How organisms grow.

• **Genotype:** The genetic makeup, i.e. the genetic constitution, of individual organisms (microbial strains).

• **Phenotype:** The set of observable characteristics of a microbe that results from the interaction of the genotype with the environment.

• **Phylogeny:** The evolutionary development and diversification of microorganisms. Sometimes referred to as *phylogenesis*, phylogeny is important as it facilitates the identification of new discovered microorganisms, but also because it helps us see the relationships between different microbes. Phylogeny is studied using genetics, molecular as well as evolutionary biology.

3

The study of Microbiology enables the treatment and prevention of diseases caused by microorganisms such as bacteria, viruses, protozoa, and fungi. Besides this, microbiology is also central to industries such as pharmaceuticals, genetics, nutrition and mining. It is important to consider that the study of microbiology is crucial for a great variety of professions - from medicine, nursing, pharmaceuticals and clinical lab technology, to environmental engineering, brewing and winemaking.

Among other things, you will discover:

- The common characteristics of microorganisms.
- How microbes are different from one another.
- The processes quintessential to microbial life.
- The diversity of microbial life.
- The ways in which microbes impact our lives.
- How microbes are identified and classified.
- The clinical manifestations, diagnostics, and virulence factors of clinically significant microbes.
- How diseases caused by microbes are treated.
- The types, structure, and replication of viruses.
- The functioning of the different parasites and the diseases they cause.
- The types of fungi and their implications for humans and plants.
- And much more!

The ultimate aim of this book is to kick-start your understanding of microbial life. It is tailored toward the lifelong learner and explorer. It can also be used by students dipping into the subject, along with their core microbiology text - or as a convenient review tool!

It is important to remember that there are always new horizons to explore with your microbial knowledge. Microbiology is an ever-evolving subject and scientists make new discoveries all the time. I hope that you enjoy this introduction to microbiology and that it marks the beginning of a lifelong exploration and appreciation for the invisible world we cannot see.

Best wishes,

Dr. Joshua Larsen

Section 2: Discovering Microbial Life

Microorganisms, as the name suggests, are microscopic organisms that play a huge role in our lives. In this section – before taking closer look at microbial morphology, classification and growth – we will explore exactly what microorganisms are and how they came into being.

1. WHAT ARE MICROORGANISMS?

Microorganisms or microbes comprise a diverse group of organisms. They are defined as living, microscopic organisms – which can be single-celled or multicellular – that typically require a microscope to be seen. Microbiology (the study of microorganisms) began with Antonie van Leeuwenhoek, a Dutch scientist who discovered microorganisms in 1674 with the use of a microscope.

From an evolutionary perspective, there are three main types of microorganisms.

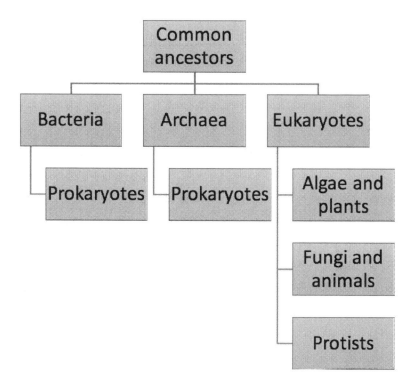

Bacteria: Bacteria are a group of unicellular organisms that are, despite the fact that there are many different kinds, broadly categorized as being either *Gram-positive* or *Gram-Gram-negative*.

Archaea: Archaea, also called archaebacteria, are a group of unicellular organisms that have evolved alongside bacteria. Despite this, they are different from bacteria in certain aspects of their chemical structure. Many archaea are *extremophiles*, which means that they thrive in extreme environments - in very acidic and very hot conditions. Archaebacteria are more closely related to eukaryotes than they are to bacteria.

Eukaryotic microorganisms: Eukaryotic microbes comprise a diverse group of organisms that include algae, fungi and protists. Unlike prokaryotes, which do not have a distinct nucleus, nor specialized organelles, all eukaryotic microorganisms have a nucleus, containing genetic material in the form of chromosomes, and membrane-bound organelles. Eukaryotes include all living organisms, apart from eubacteria and archaebacteria.

Viruses: Viruses, which include prions and sub-viral particles, typically consist of a nucleic acid molecule in a protein coat. In other words, viruses are made up of genetic material enclosed by a viral coat. This group however does not possess the machinery for producing proteins and catalyzing reactions. Viruses are smaller than bacteria and must infect and 'hijack' machinery from a host cell in order to survive and duplicate.

Despite the wide range of microorganisms, the study of microbiology typically encompasses the study of bacteria and archaea exclusively. This is because the studies of other microorganisms are typically considered specialties *per se.* The study of viruses for example, falls under virology, the study of algae under phycology, and the study of fungi is entitled mycology.

2. THE EVOLUTIONARY TREE OF LIFE

Early on when the earth was formed roughly four billion years ago, primitive cells diverged in two different directions – leading to bacteria and archaea. Each of these 'branches', as depicted in the evolutionary tree of life, was most likely accustomed to different environmental conditions, which in turn gave rise to the differences in their structural foundation and metabolic specialization.

Bacteria and Archaea – Structural Differences		
	Bacteria	**Archaea**
Metabolism specialization	Endospores Chlorophyll photosynthesis	Can grow above 100°C
Cell wall	Peptidoglycan	No peptidoglycan
Lipid Membrane	Ester-linked	Ether-linked
Enzymes for transcription of nucleic acids	One enzyme with 4 subunits	One enzyme with 8 – 10 subunits
Enzymes for protein synthesis	70S ribosome	70S ribosome

Early phototrophic organisms used sunlight as energy, but it was the arrival of oxygenic phototrophic organisms (organisms that produced oxygen as a waste product) that really kick-started evolutionary diversity on earth. After a few hundred million years, oxygen levels in the atmosphere eventually rose to levels high enough for aerobic microorganisms to evolve. However, oxygen was toxic for many anaerobic microorganisms, which meant that they either had to develop mechanisms that allowed them to tolerate oxygen presence, or they would be restricted to living in locations without oxygen.

As the levels of oxygen in the atmosphere rose over the ensuing years, microorganisms with organelles (the eukaryotes) evolved. Eventually, this gave rise to the new taxon that we know as Eukarya or Eukaryota.

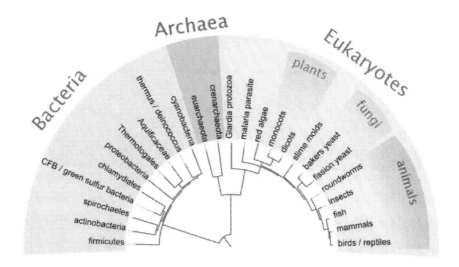

The fundamental difference and main distinguishing feature between eukaryotes and prokaryotes (which includes bacteria and archaea) is the presence of a nucleus and of membrane-bound organelles.

Eukaryotes however, are in many ways more similar to organisms belonging to the Archaea branch. In fact, eukaryotes evolved from an archaeal ancestor that engulfed but failed to destroy a bacterial cell. This resulted in a symbiotic relationship called *endosymbiosis*. It was this symbiotic relationship that gave rise to Eukaryotes.

Endosymbiosis

While there is still debate surrounding the exact order in which the following events unraveled, the majority of evolutionary biologists are generally in agreement that the following took place:

1. An aerobic bacterial cell was engulfed, eventually becoming a mitochondrion.
2. Formation of a nuclear membrane around the chromosome of the cell.
3. A cyanobacteria was engulfed, eventually becoming a chloroplast, which in turn gave rise to algae and eventually plants.
4. Formation of membrane-bound organelles.

The 'merging' of two separate organisms in order to form a single organism, is referred to as *symbiogenesis* or *endosymbiotic* theory. Symbiogenesis, as illustrated in the diagram below, represents one of the evolutionary theories for the origin of eukaryotic cells and it has gained widespread popularity in recent times.

The endosymbiotic theory proposes that the symbiotic consortiums of prokaryotes were the ancestors of eukaryotes. It states that eukaryotes evolved during the time when prokaryotes were engulfed and incorporated inside larger prokaryotes. They then eventually developed to become mitochondria, chloroplasts, and potentially also grew to become several other key organelles. According to the theory, a prokaryotic cell capable of engulfing other prokaryotic cells engulfed an aerobic bacterial cell. But instead of digesting the autotrophic bacterium, the bacteria remained, benefiting the host cell by helping to generate additional energy in the form of ATP, and by removing harmful oxygen molecules. The host cell in turn provided protection as well as a steady environment inside which the bacterium could live. In other words, they formed a mutually beneficial symbiotic relationship in which they were dependent upon another to varying degrees. This interdependence slowly grew and the bacterium eventually evolved into being a mitochondrion. It is this process (endosymbiosis) by which these prokaryotes evolved to form the first eukaryotic cells.

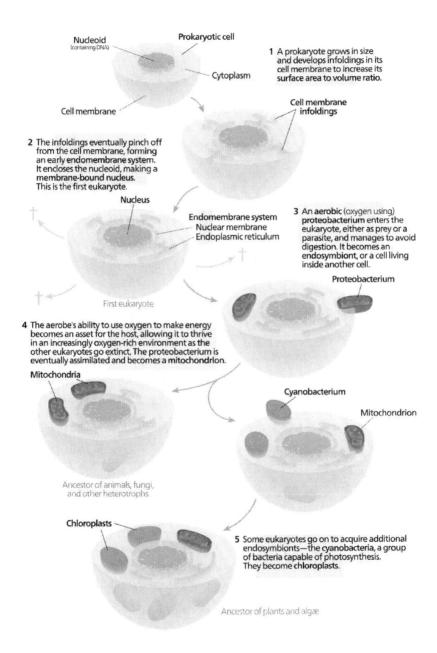

The result of this evolutionary development is what we know as the *tree of life*. However, determining the evolutionary history of organisms can be challenging. One reason for this is that bacteria and archaea can transfer their genetic code in different ways, horizontally or vertically.

Vertical Gene Transfer

Vertical gene transfer or vertical transmission is the transfer of genetic material from a 'parent' cell to a 'daughter' cell. In bacteria and archaea, this is achieved through **cell division.** During cell division, replication errors may occur which are transferred from the parent genome to the daughter cells. This can lead to mutations that can persist throughout the generations that follow.

Horizontal Gene Transfer

Horizontal gene transfer (HGT), which is synonymous with lateral gene transfer (LGT), is the incorporation of whole genes or sections of DNA in the genome from an external, 'outside' source. It is the movement or transfer of genetic material between unicellular and/or multicellular organisms. This occurs in a number of ways, including through mechanisms such as transformation and transfection. HGT can lead to genes from entirely different and unrelated species being incorporated into the same genome.

Phylogenetic Tree of Life

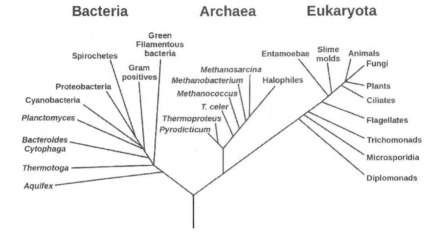

Section 3: Bacteriology – All About Bacteria

In this section we will explore Gram stain, bacterial shapes and structures (bacterial morphology), as well as the metabolic, genetic and immunologic characteristics of bacterial cells.

1. GRAM STAIN

Gram stain, sometimes also referred to as the Gram's method, is a staining technique that is used primarily to identify bacteria. During Gram Stain, a violet stain is applied to the bacteria, followed by a decolorizing agent and a red stain.

Gram Staining Procedure

Process of test	Appearance of Cells
Step 1: Begin with heat fixed cells	
Step 2: Flood slide with crystal violet dye for 1 min.	
Step 3: Add iodine solution for 1 min.	
Step 4: Wash slide with alcohol for 20sec.	
Step 5: Counter stain with safranin.	

The four simple steps of Gram stain are as follows:

1. Apply violet (bluish) dye and wait for 60 seconds.
2. Wash off with water, then with iodine solutions, and wait for another 60 seconds.
3. Wash off with water and pour on 95% alcohol (the decolorizing agent).
4. Counterstain with safranin, a red dye, and wash off with water after 30 seconds.

Those bacteria whose walls retain the violet (bluish) dye are 'Gram-positive'. Those bacteria that appear red as the second dye, not having retained the first dye, are said to be 'Gram-Gram-negative.' This differences in color results from differences in the cell walls of the bacteria.

Gram Positive Cell Wall		Gram Negative Cell Wall	
Effect of Step	Effect on Cell Wall	Effect of Step	Effect on Cell Wall
Step 1: Cell wall remains clear.		Step 1: Cell wall remains clear.	
Step 2: Peptidoglycan cell wall is flooded with crystal violet and appears purple.		Step 2: Cell wall is stained purple from the crystal violet dye.	
Step 3: A crystal violet – iodine complex is formed within the peptidoglycan cell wall trapping the purple stain.		Step 3: A crystal violet-iodine complex is formed but does not adhere to the cell wall due to the thin layer of peptidoglycan.	
Step 4: The crystal violet – iodine complex is trapped with the peptidoglycan cell wall and doesn't wash out.		Step 4: The crystal violet – iodine structure is washed out of the thin peptidoglycan layer.	
Step 5: As the peptidoglycan cell wall remains stained purple the red safranin has no effect.		Step 5: The red safranin stains the washed gram negative cells.	

Gram-Positive and Gram Gram-Negative Bacterial Cell Wall

Gram-positive and gram Gram-negative organisms both have more than one layer separating their cytoplasm from the external, extracellular environment.

The layer external to the bacterial plasma membrane, present in both Gram-positive and gram Gram-negative bacteria, is the **peptidoglycan layer**. The peptidoglycan layer, also called murein, is a polymer composed of disaccharides and amino acids, which forms the cell wall.

The amino acid chains of the peptidoglycan bind to amino acids from other nearby chains, forming a rigid and strong cell wall structure. This linkage is catalyzed by the bacterial enzyme **transpeptidase**, which is found in the inner cytoplasmic membrane.

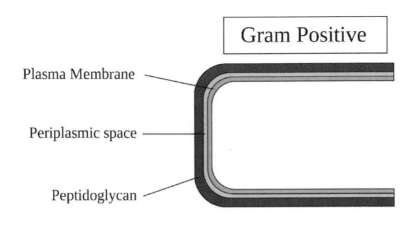

Gram Positive

Plasma Membrane

Periplasmic space

Peptidoglycan

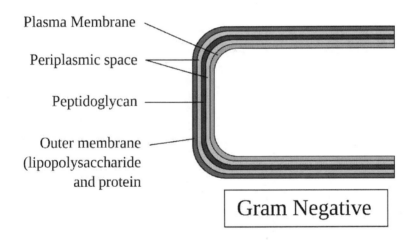

Plasma Membrane

Periplasmic space

Peptidoglycan

Outer membrane
(lipopolysaccharide
and protein

Gram Negative

The main difference between Gram-positive cell walls and Gram Gram-negative cell walls is that Gram-positive bacterial cell walls are thick - comprised of substantial cross-linking between neighboring amino acid chains. Gram Gram-negative bacterial cell walls are thin, containing only a thin layer between the outer membrane and the cytoplasmic membrane, with comparatively little cross-linking.

- **Gram-Positive Bacterial Cell Wall:**

The Gram-positive bacterial cell wall is composed of an outer layer of complexly cross-linked **peptidoglycan** (number 2), **lipoteichoic acid** (number 5), **teichoic acid, polysaccharides,** and other **proteins**. Of these, teichoic acid acts as an antigenic determinant or epitope, i.e. the site at the antigen molecule to which the antibody attaches itself. The inner surface of the Gram-positive bacterial cell wall touches the **cytoplasmic membrane** (number 1), which is composed of a lipid bilayer and contains **phospholipid** (number 3) and **proteins** (number 4). Unlike the plasma membrane in animal cells, the plasma membrane in bacteria contains no cholesterol or sterols.

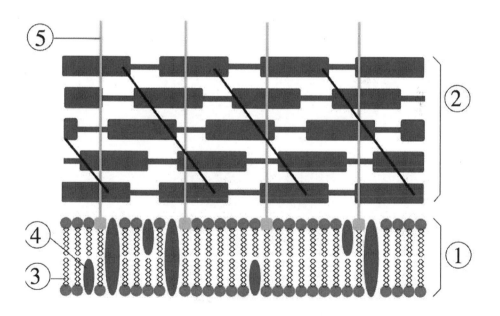

- **Gram Gram-Negative Bacterial Cell Wall:**

The Gram Gram-negative bacterial cell wall is similar to the Gram-positive bacterial cell wall in that it has a cytoplasmic membrane that is enclosed by a **peptidoglycan layer** (number 5). However, it differs from the Gram-positive bacterial cell in that it also has an **outer cytoplasmic cell membrane** (number 3). Both the **inner cytoplasmic membrane** (number 1) and the outer cytoplasmic membrane contain a **phospholipid bilayer** (number 4) and various **proteins** (number 7). The outer layer however differs in that it contains as **lipopolysaccharides or LPS** (number 8) on its external side. LPS, also known as endotoxins or lipoglycans, are large molecules comprising a polysaccharide and a lipid composed of O-antigen that elicit strong immune responses in animals.

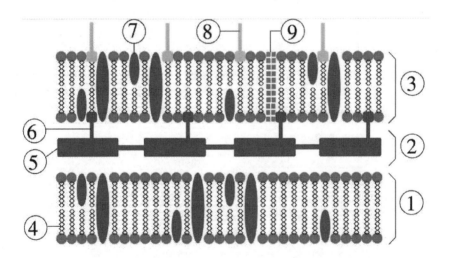

Compared to the Gram-positive bacterial cell wall, the **peptidoglycan layer** (number 5) of the Gram Gram-negative bacterial cell wall is significantly thinner and lies inside a gel-filled space containing proteins and enzymes, called the **periplasmic space** (number 2).

Furthermore, unlike the Gram-positive bacterial cell wall, the Gram Gram-negative bacterial cell wall does not contain teichoic acid, but instead has a lipoprotein called **murein lipoprotein** (number 6), alongside other proteins, including porins (number 9). Porins are beta barrel proteins that span the width of the cellular membrane, through which small ions and molecules can diffuse. The murein lipoprotein springs from the peptidoglycan layer and extends into the outer cytoplasmic cell membrane, binding the latter to the former.

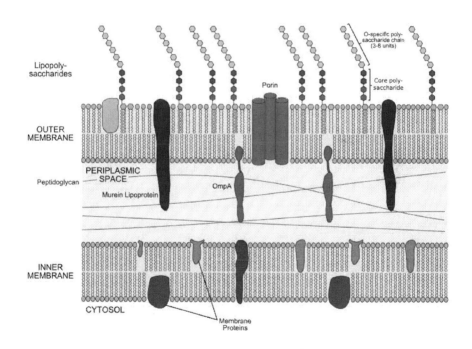

Gram-Positive and Gram Gram-Negative Cells: An Overview

Gram-Positive Cells	Gram Gram-Negative Cells
Retains violet dye, stains blue or purple.	Decolorizes, but retains safranin counterstain, stains pink or red.
Comprises two layers: 1. An inner cytoplasmic membrane 2. An outer (thick & multi-layered) peptidoglycan layer (60 – 100% peptidoglycan)	Comprises three layers: 1. An inner cytoplasmic membrane 2. A (thin & single-layered) peptidoglycan layer (5 – 10% peptidoglycan) 3. An outer membrane that contains lipopolysaccharides (LPS)
Cell wall is smooth and 20 – 30 nm thick	Cell wall is wavy and 8 – 12 nm thick
Vulnerable to lysozyme (high cell wall disruption), penicillin and sulfonamide attacks, more susceptible to antibiotics	Resistant to lysozyme (low cell wall disruption), penicillin and sulfonamide attacks, less resistant to antibiotics
No periplasmic space	Contains a periplasmic space between membranes
No porin proteins	Contains porin protein channel(s)

No endotoxins (except for Listeria monocytogenes) – virtually no LPS	Contains Endotoxins (LPS), Lipid A – high LPS content
Many contain teichoic acids	No teichoic acids
Produces primarily exotoxins	Produces primarily endotoxins
Mesosome is more prominent	Mesosome is less prominent
Two rings in basal body	Four rings in basal body
High resistance to physical disruption	Low resistance to physical disruption
High susceptibility to anionic detergents	Low susceptibility to anionic detergents
High resistance to sodium azide	Low resistance to sodium azide
High resistance to drying	Low resistance to drying

As a result of these differences, Gram Gram-negative and Gram-positive bacteria interact in different ways to their external environment. Due to the complex pattern and thickness of the peptidoglycan layer of Gram-positive bacteria, the Gram-positive cell wall does not block diffusion of low molecular weight compounds. This means that such substances (including antibiotics, detergents, and dyes) can pass through the cell wall. The cell walls of Gram Gram-negative cells however, which contain lipopolysaccharides, are able to block the diffusion of such molecules. This is why Gram Gram-negative cells are resistant to lysozyme and penicillin attacks – because antibiotics and chemicals that try to attack the peptidoglycan cell wall are unable to pass through.

During the Gram stain however, the violet (bluish) dye of the stain becomes trapped in the thick cell wall of Gram-positive cells, which results in a (positive) blue stain. In Gram Gram-negative bacteria, the outer cell membrane that is high in lipid is dissolved by alcohol, which clears the violet (bluish) stain, and allows safranin (red) counterstaining.

2. BACTERIAL SHAPES AND STRUCTURES

Bacterial morphology is the study of the shapes of bacteria. There are three basic bacterial shapes, which are *coccus* (spherical), *bacillus* (rod-shaped) and *spirillum* (twisted). Pleomorphic bacteria – i.e. bacteria that lack a distinct shape – can assume many different shapes.

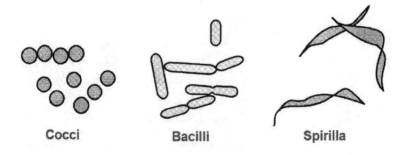

Cocci   Bacilli   Spirilla

1. **Cocci:** spherical.

2. **Bacilli:** rod-shaped; short bacilli bacteria are called cocobacilli and those that come in pairs are referred to as diplococci.
3. **Spirillum:** spiral-shaped, S-shaped, or comma-shaped.
4. **Pleomorphic:** no distinct shape.

Other (less common) shapes include:

1. **Spirochaete**: corkscrew-shaped.
2. **Vibrios**: comma-shaped.
3. **Chain of cocci.**
4. **Cluster of cocci.**
5. **Pair of cocci.**
6. **Chain of bacilli**

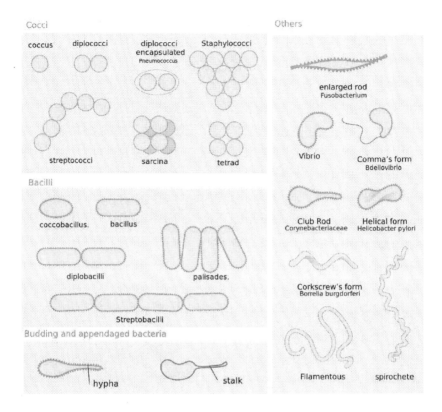

In humans, there are generally six Gram-positive bacteria that cause disease, with every other one being Gram Gram-negative. Of these six disease-causing Gram-positive bacteria, **two are cocci** and **four are bacilli**.

2 Gram-positive cocci

1. Staphylococcus forms clusters of cocci.
2. Streptococcus forms strips of cocci.

4 Gram-positive bacilli

3. Bacillus forms spores.
4. Clostridium forms spores.
5. Corynebacterium does not produce spores.
6. Listeria does not produce spores.

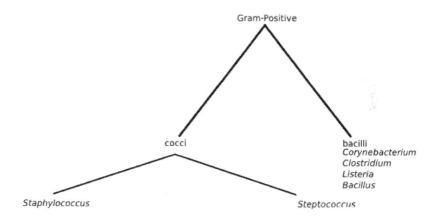

Of the Gram-negative organisms in humans, there is only one group of cocci bacteria and only one spiral-shaped group, with the rest being pleomorphic or Gram-negative rods:

1. Neisseria (diplococcus) – cocci.
2. Spirochetes – spiral.

Exceptions:

- **Mycobacteria:** This is a genus of aerobic, slightly Gram-positive and acid-fast bacteria or Actinobacteria, which occur as slightly straight or curved rods. The genus includes disease-causing pathogens such as those responsible for tuberculosis (*Mycobacterium tuberculosis*) and leprosy (*Mycobacterium leprae*).

- **Spirochetes:** Worm-like, spiral-shaped Gram-negative cells, which are too small to be seen with a typical microscope. Because of this, a special darkfield microscope must be used.

- **Mycoplasma/Spirochetes:** This is a group of small, typically disease-causing bacteria that lack a cell wall. Because they only have a simple cell membrane, they are neither Gram-positive nor Gram-negative.

Bacterial Structures of the Cytoplasm

Bacteria are prokaryotic cells. Within the cytoplasm of the bacteria, there is **bacterial DNA** – which typically comprises a single circle of double-stranded DNA, **plasmids** – smaller genetic structures that can replicate independently of the chromosomes and which typically contain antibiotic resistance genes, and **ribosomes** – composed of RNA and proteins and which comprise two subunits - a large subunit (50S) and a small subunit (30S).

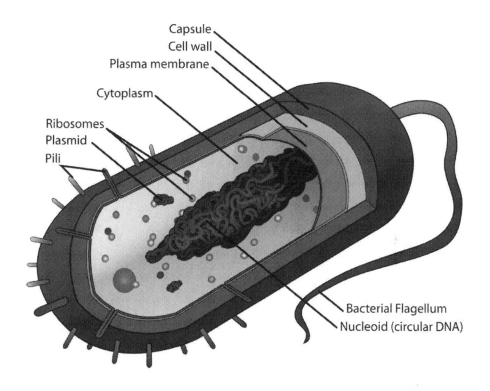

Capsule
Cell wall
Plasma membrane
Cytoplasm
Ribosomes
Plasmid
Pili
Bacterial Flagellum
Nucleoid (circular DNA)

3. BACTERIAL METABOLISM

Metabolism refers to the biochemical reactions that occur within a cell, organism, or in the case of bacterial metabolism, within a bacterium. Bacteria can be further classified into groups according to their metabolic properties – i.e. how they deal with oxygen, how they deal with their carbon and energy source, as well as according to the end products that they produce.

How Bacteria Deal With Oxygen

The way in which bacteria deal with oxygen plays a significant role in their classification. This is because molecular oxygen is extremely reactive, able to form O2- superoxide (one electron); H2O2, hydrogen peroxide (two electrons); and OH-, a hydroxyl radical (three electrons), as it takes in electrons. Unless broken down, all three products are toxic.

There are three enzymes that different bacteria possess that are able to break down these oxygen products:

- **Peroxidase** – breaks down hydrogen peroxide.
- **Catalase** – also breaks down hydrogen peroxide in the following reaction:

$$H_2O_2 + H_2O_2 \xrightarrow{\text{Catalase}} 2H_2O + O_2$$

$$H_2O_2 + H_2O_2 \xrightarrow{\text{CAT}} 2H_2O + O_2$$

- **Superoxide dismutase** – breaks down the superoxide radical:

$$2O_2^- + 2H^+ \xrightarrow{\text{Superoxide Dismutase}} O_2 + H_2O_2$$

$$\text{O}_2\text{·-} + \text{O}_2\text{·-} + 2\text{H}^+ \xrightarrow{\text{SOD}} \text{O}_2 + \text{H}_2\text{O}_2$$

Oxygen Requirements for Bacteria

Bacteria can be classified into groups according to their oxygen requirements. A bacterium's oxygen requirements are reflective of the mechanism it uses to satisfy its energy needs.

1. **Obligate aerobes:** Obligate aerobes (number 1 in the diagram below) require O2 for growth and use O2 as a final electron acceptor in aerobic respiration.
2. **Obligate anaerobes:** Obligate anaerobes, sometimes called aerophobes (number 2 in the diagram below), do not require O2 as a nutrient and are in fact poisoned by O2. Instead, obligate anaerobic prokaryotes survive by fermentation, anaerobic respiration, bacterial photosynthesis, or by the process of methanogenesis.
3. **Facultative anaerobes:** Facultative anaerobes or facultative aerobes (number 3 in the diagram below) are organisms that can switch between aerobic and anaerobic types of metabolism. In other words, they can metabolize energy aerobically and anaerobically. Under aerobic conditions (in the presence of O2), they live by aerobic respiration, and under anaerobic conditions, they grow by fermentation or anaerobic

respiration. While they have the faculty of being anaerobic, they prefer aerobic conditions.

4. **Microaerophilic:** Microaerophilic bacteria (number 4 in the diagram below), require oxygen as they cannot ferment or respire anaerobically, but are poisoned by high concentrations of oxygen.

5. **Aerotolerant anaerobes:** Aerotoleran anaerobes are bacteria that live using exclusively anaerobic (fermentative) metabolism. Unlike obligate anaerobes however, they are insensitive to O2, i.e. they are not poisoned by O2.

A bacteria's oxygen requirements (or toxicity) can be identified by growing it in test tubes of thioglycollate broth:

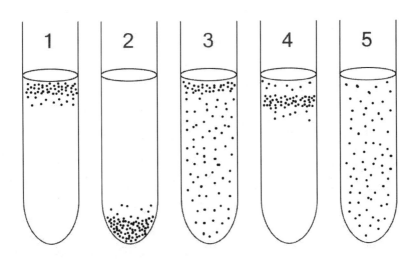

1: Obligate aerobes are found at the top of the tube where the oxygen concentration is highest.

2: Obligate anaerobes are found at the bottom of the tube where the oxygen concentration is lowest.

3: Facultative anaerobes are largely found at the top because aerobic respiration generates more ATP than either fermentation or anaerobic respiration.

4: Microaerophiles are found in the upper part of the test tube but not the very top.

5: Aerotolerant organisms are evenly spread throughout the test tube.

The spectrum of bacteria based on how they react to oxygen is as follows:

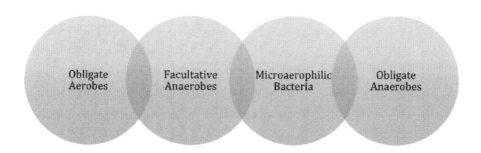

Obligate Aerobes	Facultative Anaerobes	Microaerophilic Bacteria

Cannot survive without O2.	Prefer the presence of O2 but can grow both aerobically and and anaerobically.	Can only survive in environments with very little O2.
Obligate aerobes include:	Facultative Anaerobes include:	Microaerophilic bacteria include:
<ul><li>*Nocardia*</li><li>***Bacillus cereus***</li><li>*Neisseria*</li><li>*Pseudomonas*</li><li>*Bordetella*</li><li>*Legionella*</li><li>*Brucella*</li><li>*Mycobacterium*</li><li>*Leptospira Interrogans*</li><li>*Branhamella catarrhalis*</li><li>*Burkholderia cepacia*</li><li>*Francisella tularensis*</li><li>*Spirillum minus*</li><li>*Coxiella burnetti*</li></ul>	<ul><li>*Listeria*</li><li>*Actinomyces*</li><li>*Bacillus anthracis*</li><li>*Corynebacterium*</li><li>*Staphylococcus*</li><li>*Most other Gram-negative rods*</li></ul>	<ul><li>*Enterococcus*</li><li>*some Streptococci (although some species of streptococci are facultative anaerobes)*</li><li>*Helicobacter pylori*</li><li>*Spirochetes*</li><li>*Treponema*</li><li>*Borrelia*</li><li>*Leptospira (except Leptospira interrogans)*</li><li>*Campylobacter*</li></ul>

Obligate Anaerobes
Cannot survive in the presence of O2.

Obligate Anaerobes include:

- *Clostridium*
- *Bacteroides*
- *Fusobacterium*
- *Streptobacillus moniliformis*
- *Porphyromonas*
- *Prevotella*
- *Veillonella*
- *Peptostreptococcus*

How Bacteria Deal With Their Carbon and Energy Source

Some organisms, referred to as **phototrophs**, use light as an energy source, whilst others, **chemotrophs,** use chemical compounds as an energy source.

Chemotrophs are further divided into **autotrophs**, which are organisms that use inorganic chemical energy sources (e.g. ammonium and sulfide), and **heterotrophs**, which use organic carbon sources for energy.

All clinically important bacteria are referred to as
chemoheterotrophs because they use organic chemical
compounds for energy (e.g. glucose).

Oxygen Metabolism – Fermentation and Respiration

For oxygen metabolism, many bacteria use fermentation
(glycolysis). During fermentation, glucose is broken down into
pyruvic acid, which yields energy in the form of ATP. There are
different pathways that can be used to break glucose down into
pyruvate, with the most common one being the *Embden-Meyerhof-
Parnas glycolytic pathway* (EMP pathway).

Following fermentation, the pyruvate must be broken down and
the end product formed through this process (including acetone,
butyric acid, ethanol, lactic acid, propionic acid and other mixed
acids) can be used for bacteria classification.

Other bacteria, which include aerobic and facultative anaerobic
organisms, use respiration for oxygen metabolism. Respiration
includes glycolysis, the Krebs tricarboxylic-acid cyclem, as well as
the electron transport chain with oxidative phosphorylation. All
these pathways combine, forming/synthesizing ATP in the
process.

4. GRAM-POSITIVE BACTERIA

Gram-positive bacteria are bacteria that give a positive result in
the Gram stain test previously discussed. Unlike Gram-negative

bacteria, Gram-positive bacteria have a large peptidoglycan structure. Furthermore, some Gram-positive bacteria can also – when placed under stress environmental conditions – form spores that allow the bacteria to survive this exposure to extreme conditions (e.g. when the availability of carbon and nitrogen is limited). This can lead to re-infection. Bacteria capable of forming spores are referred to as spore-formers. The diagram below outlines the general phenotypic classification of Gram-positive bacteria.

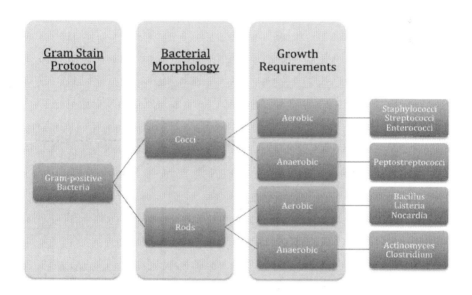

Virulence factors are molecules that are produced by pathogens – which include bacteria, fungi, protozoa and viruses – that contribute to the organism's pathogenicity. An organism's virulence is dependent upon its cell structure, exotoxins and endotoxins – which are all virulence factors.

In the following sections, we will cover bacteria genera, the major, clinically significant bacterial species, their virulence factors, clinical manifestations, as well as how they are diagnosed and treated.

Staphylococci

There are three main pathogenic species of Staphylococcus, which will be discussed in turn in this subsection: *Staphylococcus aureus, Staphylococcus epidermidis* and *Staphylococcus saprophyticus.*

1. Staphylococcus Aureus –

This Gram-positive coccal bacterium belongs to Firmicutes phylum of bacteria and is typically found on the nose, skin, and inside the respiratory tract. It can be differentiated from the other two Staphylococcus species, in that *Staphylococcus aureus* is the only one that is **coagulase positive.** Although not always pathogenic, Staphylococcus aureus is often a cause of skin infections and food poisoning. It can also cause a variety of different diseases and can infect pretty much any organ system. The diseases that can be caused by *Staphylococcus aureus* can be divided into two groups: diseases caused by the release of exotoxins, and diseases by direct organ invasion by the bacterium.

Clinical Manifestations	Diagnostics	Virulence Factors	Treatment
STAPHYLOCOCCUS AUREUS			

Exotoxin Dependent:	Gram Stain:	Protective:	1. Penicillinase-resistant penicillins such as methicillin or naficillan
1. Enterotoxin – gastroenteritis (food poisoning): rapid onset and recovery **2. Toxic shock syndrome, caused by the release of *TSST-1* – symptoms of which include high fever, nausea and vomiting, diarrhea, rash, hypotension, and desquamation of palms and soles** **3. Exfoliatin – scalded skin syndrome (in children)** **Diseases**	1. Gram (+), reveals Gram-positive, clustered cocci/cocci in grape-like clusters **Culture:** 2. β-hemolytic 3. Produces a golden, yellow pigment with sheep blood **Metabolic:** 4. Catalase (+) 5. **Coagulase (+)** 6. Facultative	1. Microcapsule 2. Protein A: binds IgG 3. Coagulase: fibrin formation around organism 4. Hemolysins 5. Leukocidins 6. Penicillinase **Tissue-Destroying:** 1. Hyaluronidase 2. Lipase 3. Staphylokinase	2. If the bacterium is methicillin-resistant, treat with Vancomycin 3. Clindamycin

resulting from Direct Organ Invasion: 1. Pneumonia 2. Meningitis, Cerebritis, Brain Abscess 3. Osteomyelitis (in children) – inflammation of the bone or bone marrow; typically due to infection 4. Acute endocarditis 5. Septic arthritis 6. Skin infections 7. Bacteremia / Sepsis 8. Urinary tract infection	anaerobe		

2. Staphylococcus Epidermidis

Staphylococcus epidermidis – which typically doesn't cause disease – is naturally found on our body (particularly on the skin and on mucous membranes), where it forms part of its cloud of microbes. The bacterium however, is a routine skin contaminant of blood cultures – infection typically occurs when a needle, Foley urine catheter or IV line covered with Staphylococcus epidermidis passes through the skin. Besides this, Staphylococcus epidermidis also has a polysaccharide capsule, which permits adherence to prosthetic materials that can lead to infections of the prosthetic devices of the body.

Clinical Manifestations	Diagnostics	Virulence Factors	Treatment
STAPHYLOCOCCUS EPIDERMIDIS			
Nosocomial Infections: **1. Prosthetic joints** **2. Prosthetic heart valves** **3. Sepsis from intravenous lines** **4. Urinary tract**	**Gram Stain:** 1. Gram (+), reveals Gram-positive, clustered cocci **Metabolic:** 2. Catalase	**Protective:** 1. Polysaccharide capsule (adheres to various prosthetic devices) 2. Highly resistant to	Vancomycin, because it's resistant to various other antibiotics

infection	(+)	antibiotics	
Skin contamination in blood cultures	3. Coagulase (-) 4. Facultative anaerobe		

3. Staphylococcus Saprophyticus

Secondary only to *E coli, Staphylococcus saprophyticus* constitutes the leading cause of urinary tract infections in young women that are sexually active.

Clinical Manifestations	Diagnostics	Virulence Factors	Treatment
STAPHYLOCOCCUS SAPROPHYTICUS			

Urinary tract infection in sexually active females	Gram Stain: 1. Gram (+), reveals Gram-positive, clustered cocci Culture: 2. γ-hemolytic Metabolic: 3. Catalase (+) 4. **Coagulase (-)** 5. Facultative anaerobe		Penicillin

Streptococci

Streptococci, like staphylococci, are Gram-positive and responsible for various different human diseases. Differentiation between the two however is necessary in order to prescribe the correct antibiotic. There are two ways in which one can differentiate streptococci from staphylococci. Firstly, by looking at the Gram stain, streptococci line up like a strip, whereas staphylococci form clusters. Secondly, by using the enzyme catalase (streptococci does not possess the enzyme catalase, whereas staphylococci do).

There are five main pathogenic species of Streptococci that will be outlined and discussed in this section: *Streptococcus Pyrogenes* (Group A), *Streptococcus agalactiae* (Group B), *Enterococci* (Group D), *Streptococcus pneumonia, Steptococcus agalactiae* and *Streptococcus viridans*.

1. Streptococcus Pyogenes (Group A)

Also referred to as Group A *Beta-Hemolytic Streptococci*, *Streptococcus Pyogenes* can cause scarlet fever, rheumatic fever, strep throat and post-streptococcal glomerulonephritis. Like the majority of the other bacteria species belonging to streptococci, *Streptococcus Pyogenes* is clinically important in human diseases. It possesses the **Lancefield group A antigen** and is thus also called Group A streptococcus.

Clinical Manifestations	Diagnostics	Virulence Factors	Treatment
STREPTOCOCCUS PYOGENES (GROUP A)			

Direct Invasion / Toxin:	Gram Stain:	1. M-protein (70 types) – adherence factor, antiphagocytic, antigenic (i.e. it induces antibodies that can result in phagocytosis)	1. Penicillin G
1. Pharyngitis (red, swollen tonsils and pharynx, purulent exudates on tonsils, fever, swollen lymph nodes)	**1. Gram (+), cocci in chains** **Culture:** 2. Inhibited by bacitracin		2. Penicillin V 3. Erythromycin
2. Sepsis **3. Skin infections (folliculitis, cellulitis, impetigo, necrotizing fasciitis)**	3. β-hemolytic (streptolysin – O – oxygen labile, antigenic; – S – oxygen stable, non-antigenic)	2. Lipoteichoic acid (adherence factor) 3. Steptokinase	4. Penicillinase-resistant penicillin (in skin infections where staphylococci might be responsible)
4. Scarlet fever (fever and scarlet red rash on body)	**Metabolic:** 4. Catalase (-)	4. Hyaluronidase	Following rheumatic fever, patients are placed on continuous prophylaxis antibiotics, so as to prevent repeat infection that could
5. Toxic shock syndrome	5. Microaerophilic	5. DNAase 6. Anti-C5a peptidase	
Antibody-mediated: **6. Rheumatic fever (fever, myocarditis, arthritis,**			

migratory polyarthritis, chorea, rash, subcutaneous nodules)			otherwise lead to another rheumatic fever.
7. Acute post-streptococcal glomerulonephrit is (tea-colored urine following pharynx infection or streptococcal skin)			If heart valve complicatio ns occur, prophylaxis antibiotics are needed before certain procedures (such as dental work) are performed, as there is a high risk of bacterial endocarditis .
			Addition of clindamycin should be considered for invasive

			streptococcus pyogenes infections, such as necrotizing fasciitis or streptococcal toxic shock syndrome.

2. Streptococcus agalactiae (Group B)

Many pregnant women carry *Streptococcus agalactiae* as part of the normal flora in their vagina. It is an asymptomatic colonizer of the human GI tract in roughly 30% of adults and pregnant women. Despite being a typically harmless, commensal bacterium, Streptococcus agalactiae can nevertheless cause severe invasive infections.

Clinical Manifestations	Diagnostics	Virulence Factors	Treatment
STREPTOCOCCUS AGALACTIAE (GROUP B)			
1. Neonatal meningitis 2. Neonatal	Gram stain: (of urine or CSF) 1. Gram (+),		Penicillin G

pneumonia	chains		
3. Neonatal sepsis	**Culture:** (of CSF, urine or blood)		
	2. β-hemolytic		
	Metabolic:		
	3. Catalase (-)		
	4. Facultative anaerobe		

3. Enterococci (Group D)

The enterococci are colonizers of the human intestines and are typically considered part of the natural bowel flora. Enterococci are nevertheless also clinically significant in causing human diseases such as urinary tract infections, biliary tract infections, bacteremia and subacute bacterial endocarditis.

Clinical Manifestations	Diagnostics	Virulence Factors	Treatment

ENTEROCOCCI (GROUP D)

1. Subacute bacterial endocarditis 2. Biliary tract infections 3. Urinary tract infections	**Gram stain:** 1. Gram (+), chains **Culture:** 2. Bile, sodium chloride 3. α,β,γ-hemolytic **Metabolic:** 4. Catalase (-) 5. Facultative anaerobe	Extracellular dextran helps them bind to heart valves (high intrinsic resistance)	1. Ampicillin, combined with aminoglycosides in endocarditis 2. Resistant to penicillin G 3. Emerging resistance to vancomycin

4. Streptococcus pneumonia (pneumococci)

Streptococcus pneumonia, which does not contain any Lancefield antigens, is a principal cause of otitis media in children, of meningitis in adults, and the primary cause of pneumonia in adults. Because there are 83 different capsule types (the major virulence factor of which is polysaccharide capsule), this means that having gone through one infection only gives you immunity to one capsule type.

Clinical Manifestations	Diagnostics	Virulence Factors	Treatment
STREPTOCOCCUS PNEUMONIA (PNEUMOCOCCI)			
1. Pneumonia **2. Meningitis** **3. Sepsis** **4. Otitis media (in children)** **Toxins – secretes pneumolysins that bind cholesterol of host-cell membranes, yet its actual effect is unknown**	**Gram stain:** 1. Gram (+), diplococci **Culture:** 2. Does not grow in presence of optochin and bile 3. α-hemolytic **Metabolic:** 4. Catalase (-) 5. Facultative	Capsule (83 serotypes)	1. Penicillin G (IM) 2. Erythromycin 3. Ceftriaxone 4. Vaccine: against the 23 most common capsular antigens

| | anaerobe

Positive (+) Quellung test: (encapsulated bacteria) – quellung reaction is the technique used to detect encapsulated bacteria such as *H. influenzae* and *S. pneumoniae* | | |

5. Streptococcus viridans

Streptococcus viridans form part of the natural oral flora and are typically found in the GI tract, nasopharynx and the gingival crevices. They are Gram-positive, microaerophilic (i.e. requiring little free oxygen), and are typically isolated from abscesses.

Clinical Manifestations	Diagnostics	Virulence Factors	Treatment
STREPTOCOCCUS VIRIDANS			

1. Subacute bacterial endocarditis **2. Dental cavities – caused by** *Streptococcus mutans* **3. Brain or liver abscesses – caused by** *Streptococcus intermedius group*	**Gram stain:** 1. Gram (+), chains **Culture:** 2. Resistant to optochin 3. α-hemolytic (green) **Metabolic:** 4. Catalase (-) 5. Facultative anaerobe		Penicillin G

Spore-Forming Rods

As discussed earlier, there are six clinically important Gram-positive bacteria: two are cocci and four are rods (bacilli). Of these, two rods are spore-formers, whereas the other two are not. In the previous subsection, we have discussed the two Gram-positive cocci (**staphylococci** and **streptococci**). In this subsection, we will go on to outline and explore the two spore-forming rods: **bacillus** and **clostridium.**

Both bacillus and clostridium can cause disease through the release of potent exotoxins, but they differ biochemically by their relationship to oxygen – bacillus are aerobic whereas clostridium grow anaerobically.

BACILLUS

1. Bacillus anthracis

A unique feature of *Bacillus anthracis* is that it is the only bacterium whose capsule is composed of poly-D-glutamic acid protein – this is so as to prevent phagocytosis. Bacillus anthracis is a cause of a disease affecting herbivores, anthrax, which is a disease of sheep and cattle that typically affects the skin and the lungs. When transmitted to humans, the bacterial disease can cause severe skin ulceration or Wool-sorters' disease, a pulmonary form of anthrax caused by the inhalation or ingestion of the spores of the bacterium.

Clinical Manifestations	Diagnostics	Virulence Factors	Treatment
		BACILLUS ANTHRACIS	
Anthrax toxin (exotoxin): 3 proteins	Gram Stain: 1. Gram (+),	1. Unique protein capsule (polymer of γ-	1. Penicillin G 2.

(protective Ag (PA), edema factor (EF), lethal factor (LF))	spore-forming rods	D-glutamic acid: antiphagocytic	Erythromycin
			3. Vaccine: for high-risk individuals
	Metabolism:	2. Non-motile	
	2. Aerobe (can be facultative)	3. Virulence depends on acquiring two plasmids; one that carries the gene for protein capsule, and another that carries the gene for exotoxin	- composed of protective Ag
Anthrax: painless black vesicles; can be fatal if untreated, woolsorter's pulmonary disease, abdominal pain, vomiting and bloody diarrhea (infection results in permanent immunity if pt survives)	**Serology**		- animal vaccine composed of live strain, attenuated by loss of its protein capsule

CLOSTRIDIUM

2. Clostridium tetani

Clostridium tetani, which are introduced via wounds, are

endospores that cause tetanus – a bacterial disease characterised by rigidity, sustained contraction of skeletal muscles and spasms of voluntary muscles. *Clostridium tetani* spores – which can grow as long as there is a localized anaerobic environment such as necrotic tissue – are typically found animal feces and in the soil.

Clinical Manifestations	Diagnostics	Virulence Factors	Treatment
CLOSTRIDIUM TETANI			
Tetanospasmin: inhibits release of GABA and glycine (that are both inhibitory neurotransmitters) from nerve cells, which results in sustained muscle contraction **1. Muscle spasm** **2. Lockjaw (trismus)** **3. Risus sardonica** **4. Opisthotones (pronounced back arch)** **5. Respiratory**	**Gram Stain:** 1. Gram (+), spore-forming rods (drumstick appearance) **Metabolism:** 2. Anaerobe	Flagella (H-Ag (+))	1. Tetanus toxoid: vaccine with formalin-inactivated toxin (part of the DPT vaccine – Diphtheria, Tetanus, and Pertussis) 2. Antitoxin: human tetanus immune globulin (for those never immunized) 3. Clean the wound

| muscle paralysis | | | 4. Penicillin or metronidazole

5. Ventilatory assistance (supportive assistance) |

3. Clostridium botulinum

Clostridium botulinum is a bacterium – typically found in soil, smoked fish, canned food and honey – that produces an extremely lethal neurotoxin responsible for food poisoning that can worsen rapidly and be fatal. The neurotoxin the bacterium releases causes flaccid muscle paralyses by blocking the release of Ach (acetylcholine) from the presynaptic nerve terminals in the motor endplates and in the autonomic nervous system.

Clinical Manifestations	Diagnostics	Virulence Factors	Treatment
CLOSTRIDIUM BOTULINUM			
1. Neurotoxin: inhibits release of ACh (acetylcholine) from	**Gram stain:** 1. Gram (+), spore-forming rods	Flagella (H-Ag (+))	1. Antitoxin 2. Penicillin 3. Hyperbaric oxygen – to

peripheral nn 2. The toxin is not secreted but instead released upon death of the organism Food-borne botulism: 1. Cranial nerve palsies 2. Muscle weakness 3. Respiratory paralysis Infant botulism: 1. Constipation and 2. Flaccid paralysis	**Culture:** 2. Requires anaerobic conditions **Metabolism:** 3. Anaerobe		be administered in a high pressure chamber 4. Ventilatory assistance and intubation (supportive therapy)

4.   Clostridium perfringens or Gas Gangrene

Clostridium perfringens spores can be found in soil and food. The bacterium only grows in anaerobic conditions – e.g. conditions such as those created by dead tissue – can produce gas, as well as exotoxin enzymes that aggravate tissue destruction. There are generally two classes of infection when it comes to *Clostridium perfringens:* Firstly, cellulitis/wound infection and clostridial myonecrosis, which, if unidentified and left untreated, can be fatal.

Clinical Manifestations	Diagnostics	Virulence Factors	Treatment
CLOSTRIDIUM PERFRINGENS			
1. Alpha toxin: lecithinase (splits lecithin into phosphocholine and diglyceride) **2. Gaseous gangrene** **- cellulites / wound infection** **- clostridial myonecrosis, which can be fatal if untreated** **3. Superantigen: (spores in food) – food poisoning**	**Gram stain:** 1. Gram (+), spore-forming rods **Metabolism:** 2. Anaerobe	Non-motile	1. Radical surgery (amputation) 2. Penicillin & clindamycin 3. Hyperbaric oxygen

5. Clostridium difficile

Clostridium difficile, the bacteria responsible for antibiotic-associated pseudomembranous enterocolitis (diarrhea), is found in the intestinal tract. Such antibiotics are capable of destroying the normal flora of the intestines, which in turn enables the bacterium to superinfect the colon. *Clostridium difficile* endospores are found in hospitals and nursing homes. As the bacterium grows, it releases exotoxins – Toxin A causes diarrhea and Toxin B is cytotoxic to the colonic epithelial cells.

Clinical Manifestations	Diagnostics	Virulence Factors	Treatment
CLOSTRIDIUM DIFFICILE			
Toxin A: **1. Diarrhea** **Toxin B:** **2. Cytotoxic to the colonic epithelial cells** **Pseudomembranou s enterocolitis: antibiotic-associated diarrhea**	**Gram stain:** **1. Gram (+), spore-forming rods** **Metabolism:** 2. Anaerobe **Immunoassa y test for *C. Difficile* toxin**	Flagella (H-Ag (+))	1. Metronidazol e 2. Oral vancomycin 3. Terminate use of the responsible antibiotic

	Colonoscopy to examine the colon		

LISTERIA

6. Listeria monocytogenes

Listeria monocytogenes is a pathogenic Gram-positive motile rod bacterium that has endotoxins and which can infect the brain, spinal cord membranes and the bloodstream of the host. The bacterium, which is facultative anaerobic, meaning it can survive in the presence or absence of oxygen, is the principal cause of the bacterial infection listeriosis – a disease which primarily affects older adults, pregnant women and newborns. The bacterium can be contracted through the ingestion of unpasteurized dairy, contaminated raw milk or cheese. Besides oral ingestion, the bacterium can also be vaginally transmitted – which constitutes one of the leading causes of meningitis in newborns.

Clinical Manifestations	Diagnostics	Virulence Factors	Treatment
LISTERIA MONOCYTOGENES			
1. Neonatal	Gram Stain:	1. Flagella	1. Ampicillin

meningitis	1. Gram (+), non-spore-forming rods	(H-Ag (+))	2. Trimethoprim / Sulfamethoxazole
2. Meningitis in immuno-suppressed pts*		2. Hemolysin	
		- heat labile	
	Culture:	- antigenic	
3. Septicemia	2. Low temperature (2.5°C)		
* cell-mediated immunity protective			
** only gram (+) w/endotoxin (LPS-Lipid A) — clinical significance is ambiguous	**Metabolism:**		
	3. Catalase (+)		
	4. β-hemolysis		
	5. Facultative intracellular anaerobic parasite		

Dr. Joshua Larsen

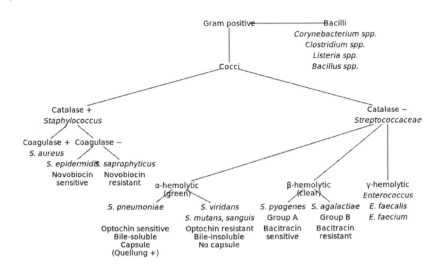

5. GRAM-NEGATIVE BACTERIA

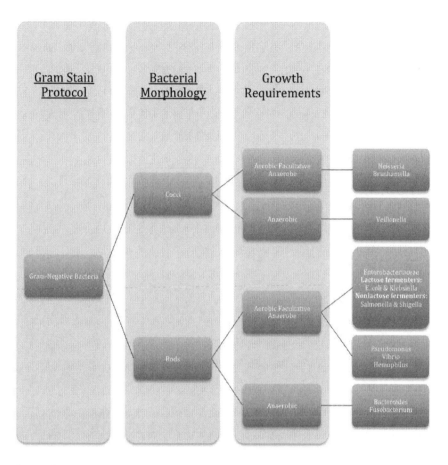

In this subsection, we will explore the pathogenic Gram-negative bacteria, that is, bacteria that do not retain the purple dye in the Gram stain test and instead appear red from the counterstain (typically safranin).

We will begin by looking at the only Gram-negative cocci bacteria, *Neisseria,* and its two species: *Neisseria meningitidis* and *Neisseria gonorrhoeae* – before covering Gram-negative rods related to the enteric tract, or 'The Enterics' for short. There are several bacterial families that fall under 'The Enterics', which include *Enterobacteriaceae, Vibrionaceae, Pseudomonadaceae* and *Bacteroidaceae.* After covering this category, we will then explore Gram-negative rods related to respiratory tract infections, in particular, those bacterial species belonging to *Hemophilus, Bordetella* and *Legionella.* Following this, we will look at Gram-negative obligate intracellular parasites, namely those bacterial species belonging to the bacterial families of *Chlamydia, Ricksettsia* and *Ehrlicihia.* Last but not least, we will cover the Gram-negative spirochete species belonging to *Treponema* and *Borrelia.*

I.   Gram-Negative Cocci

NEISSERIA

Neisseria is a kidney-bean-shaped diplococcus and the only pathogenic Gram-negative cocci. There are two pathogenic Neisseria species: *Neisseria meningitidis* and *Neisseria gonorrhoeae.*

1. Neisseria meningitidis

Neisseria meningitidis, also referred to as meningococcus, can cause meningitis and sepsis (meningococcemia). Among those at high risk of contracting *Neisseria meningitides,* which spreads via respiratory transmission (secretions), are neonates, infants between the age of 6 months and two years and army recruits. The appearance of a petechial rash, which can appear red, brown or purple, is often indicative of an invasive meningococcal infection.

Clinical Manifestations	Diagnostics	Virulence Factors	Treatment
NEISSERIA MENINGITIDIS			
1. Endotoxin: LPS **1. Meningitis – symptoms include fever, stiff neck (nuchal rigidity), vomiting, lethargy, altered mental state, petechial rash** **2. Septocemia – symptoms include fever, petechial rash, hypotension,**	**Gram Stain:** 1. Gram (-) diplococci **Culture:** (Thayer-martin VCN) 2. Grows best in a high CO_2 environment Metabolism 3. Ferments maltose and glucose 4. Facultative	1. Capsule: - 9 serotypes - A, B, C serotypes associated with meningitis 2. IgA1 protease 3. Can extract iron (Fe) 4. Pili (for adherence)	1. **Vaccine** against capsular antigens: for A, C, Y and W-135 only (not B because antibodies do not form against B) 2. **Antibiotics** - Penicillin G - Ceftriaxone (or other 3rd generation cephalosporins) - Rifampin used

waterhouse-friderichsen syndrome: bilateral hemorrhage of adrenal glands along with petechial rash and hypotension	anaerobe		prophylactically for close contact of infected individuals
3. Asymptomatic carriage in nasopharynx of humans only			

2. Neisseria gonorrhoeae

Neisseria gonorrhoeae, sometimes referred to as gonococcus, is the cause of the second most contracted STI (sexually transmitted disease): gonorrhoea. Some diseases caused by this bacterium arise in men or women exclusively, while other diseases are shared between both sexes – which include gonococcal bacteraemia and septic arthritis. In infants, *Neisseria gonorrhoeae*, which is transmitted during delivery, can lead to ophthalmia neonatorum. This is better known as Neonatal conjunctivitis, a neonatal infection which is a form of conjunctivitis. The infection can damage the cornea and lead to blindness.

Men can contract an infection with *Neisseria gonorrhoeae* through unprotected sexual transmission. Once contracted, the bacterium penetrates the mucous membrane of the urethra, which leads to urethritis (an inflammation of the urethra). This in turn leads to painful urination in some infected men, whilst others. Regardless of whether the carrier is symptomatic or asymptomatic, he can he pass the infection on to another sexual partner.

Women can likewise develop urethritis. While an infection in women is more likely to be asymptomatic, some infected women will experience purulent discharge from the urethra and a painful burning sensation when urinating. Like men however, both symptomatic and asymptomatic women can pass on the infection to their sexual partner. If the gonococcal infection reaches the cervix, the disease can progress into PID (**pelvic inflammatory disease**) – which is an infection of the Fallopian tubes (**salpingitis**), ovaries (**oophoritis**) and/or uterus (**endometritis**). Symptoms of PID include abnormal menstrual bleeding, cervical motion tenderness, fever and lower abdominal pain. Besides *Neisseria gonorrhoeae*, another major cause of PID is *Chlamydia trachomatis*.

Clinical Manifestations	Diagnostics	Virulence Factors	Treatment
NEISSERIA GONORRHOEAE			

1. Endotoxin: LPS (lipopolysaccharide)	Gram Stain:	1. Pili	1. First line
- Men: urethritis	1. Gram (-) diplococci	- Adherence (the Pili adhere to epithelial cells, which allows the bacterium to cause disease)	- 3rd generation Cephalosporins
- Women: cervical gonorrhoea, which can progress into PID	Culture: (urethral pus; the classic medium for culturing the bacterium is called the Thayer-martin VCN – vancomycin, colistin, nyastatin – media)	- Antigenic variation - Antiphagocytic: binds bacteria tightly to host cell, thus protecting it from phagocytosis	(such as ceftriaxone), to which doxycycline must be added for chlamydia and syphilis
2. No exotoxins			
3. Often asymptomatic but still infectious			2. Second line (not effective for syphilis)
- Both men and women: gonococcal bacteremia, septic arthritis – of which *Neisseria gonorrhoeae* is the most common cause	2. WBCs: Gram stain of the urethral pus will reveal small Gram-negative diplococcic within white blood cells		- Fluoroquinolones - Spectinomycin
		2. IgA1 protease	
- Neonates: opthalia neonatorum		3. Outer membrane proteins:	3. For ophthalmia neonatorum:
conjunctivitis (usually arises in first 5 days following birth)	3. Grows best in a	- Protein I:	- Erythromycin eye drops

| | high CO2 environment

Metabolism

4. Ferments only glucose (not maltose)

5. Facultative anaerobe | porin

- Protein II (opacity protein): presence associated with dark, opaque colonies for adherence | which must be given immediately following birth for prophylaxis against *Neisseria gonorrhoeae* and against *Chlamydia trachomatis* conjunctivitis

b. Infants with the disease need systemic treatment with ceftriaxone and erythromycin |

II. The Enterics: Gram-Negative Rods Related to the Enteric Tract

The Enterics – i.e. rod-shaped Gram-negative bacteria – are naturally or pathogenically present in the intestines of humans and animals. They are typically part of the normal gut flora. In this section, we will explore four taxonomic families all of which belong to the Enterics. The first is **Enterobacteriaceae**, to which belongs *Escherichia Coli, Klebsiella pneumonia, Salmonella speices and typhi* and *Shigella dysenteriae*. Also belonging to the Enterics is the family **Vibrionaceae,** where we will explore *Vibrio cholera, Campylobacter jejuni* and *Helicobacter pylori.* Lastly, we will have a closer look at the **Pseudomonadaceae,** (specifically, *Pseudomonas aeruginosa)* and at the family **Bacteroidaceae** (specifically, *Bacteroides fragilis)* – both of which also belong to the Enterics.

ENTEROBACTERIACEAE

1. Escherichia Coli

Escherichia coli, a bacterium belonging to the family Enterobacteriaceae, is naturally found in the human gastrointestinal and urinary tract. Transmitted via the fecal-oral route, migration up the urethra, aspiration of oral *Escherichia coli* and through the colonization of catheters (in hospitalized patients), *Escherichia coli* can, in the presence of virulence factors, cause a variety of diseases. The diseases caused by the bacterium include *Escherichia* diarrhea, *Escherichia coli* UTI (urinary tract infection), *Escherichia coli* meningitis, *Escherichia coli* sepsis and *Escherichia coli* pneumonia.

Clinical Manifestations	Diagnostics	Virulence Factors	Treatment
ESCHERICHIA COLI			

- Enterotoxins: 1. **LT (heat labile) – increases cAMP (which is similar to cholera toxin)** 2. **ST (heat stable): increases cGMP** 3. **Shiga-like toxin (verotoxin), which inhibits protein synthesis by inactivating the 60S ribosomal subunit** - **Newborn meningitis** - **Urinary tract infection** - **Pneumonia (hospital acquired)** - **Sepsis (hospital acquired)** - **Diarrhea:** 1. *Enterotoxigenic*	**Gram stain:** 1. Gram (-) rods **Culture:** (urine, blood, CSF on EMB or MacConkey agar) 2. Grow at 45.5°C 3. Indole (+) – makes indole from tryptophan 4. β-hemolytic **Metabolism:** 5. Catalase (+) 6. Oxidase (-) 7. Ferments	1. Fimbriae (pili): colonization factor 2. Siderophore 3. Adhesins 4. Capsule (K antigen) 5. Flagella (H antigen)	1. Cephalosporins 2. Aminoglycosides 3. Trimethoprim & sulfamethoxazole 4. Fluoroquinolones

(ETEC) – the non-invasive strain: releases LT and ST toxins and causes traveler's diarrhea 2. *Enterohemorrhagic* (EHEC) – bloody diarrhea: no fever, no pus in stool – secretes Shiga-like toxin☐ hemorrhagic that causes colitis and hemolytic uremic syndrome (*E.coli* strain O157:H7) 3. *Enteroinvasive* (EIEC): bloody diarrhea with pus in stool and fever – secretes small amounts of Shiga-like toxin	lactose 8. Facultative anaerobe		

2. Klebsiella pneumonia

Klebsiella pneumonia, which is a violent form of pneumonia that often leads to the destruction of the lung tissues, is an encapsulated, non-motile enteric. In other words, it holds 0 antigen (which is why *Klebsiella pneumonia* is said to resemble 'red-currant jelly') and no H antigen. Besides sepsis, *Klebsiella pneumonia* also causes urinary tract infections in patients with Holey catheters. This being said, hospitalized patients and alcoholics are at a higher risk of contracting *Klebsiella pneumonia*, which is often (in roughly 50% cases) accompanied by bloody sputum. Despite available antibiotic therapies, mortality rate among patients with *Klebsiella pneumonia* is high.

Clinical Manifestations	Diagnostics	Virulence Factors	Treatment
KLEBSIELLA PNEUMONIA			

1. Pneumonia, with significant lung necrosis and bloody sputum; common among alcoholics and individuals with an underlying lung disease	**Gram Stain:** 1. Gram (-) rods	1. Capsule 2. Non-motile	1. Third generation cephalosporins 2. Ciprofloxacin
	Culture: 2. EMB – Eosin methylene blue / MacConkey agar		
2. Urinary tract infection (hospital acquired)			
3. Sepsis (hospital acquired)	**Metabolism:** 3. Indole (-) 4. Ferments lactose 5. Facultative anaerobe		

SALMONELLA

Salmonella is always pathogenic and can cause four disease states in humans: firstly, carrier state (occurs in people recovering from typhoid fever after contracting *Salmonella typhi*); secondly, typhoid fever (caused by *Salmonella typhi*); thirdly, sepsis (typically caused by *Salmonella choleraesuis*) and lastly, gastroenteritis or diarrhea – which, caused by any of the different *Salmonella enteritidis* serotypes, is often accompanied by abdominal pain and nausea.

3. Salmonella Species

Salmonella is a motile, non-lactose fermenter that produces H2S (hydrogen sulfide). In contrast to the other enterics, *Salmonella* lives in the GI tracts of animals. Infection is zoonotic and occurs when food or water becomes contaminated with animal feces. Many animals, such as chickens and turtles, can carry *salmonella* – a disease that is most commonly acquired through the consumption of chicken or uncooked eggs. Like *Shigella*, *Salmonella* is never considered part of the natural intestinal flora of humans.

Clinical Manifestations	Diagnostics	Virulence Factors	Treatment
SALMONELLA SPECIES			
1. Paratyphoid fever (similar to typhoid fever) **2. Gastroenteritis (diarrhea)**	**Gram Stain:** 1. Gram (-) rods **Culture:** 2. EMB – Eosin	1. Flagella (H antigen) 2. Capsule (Vi antigen) – protects against intracellular killing	1. Ciprofloxacin 2. Ceftriaxone 3. Trimethoprim and sulfamethoxazole 4. Azithromycin

3. Sepsis 4. Osteromyelitis	methylene blue / MacConkey agar 3. H2S production **Metabolism:** 4. Catalase (+) 5. Oxidase (-) 6. Ferments glucose 7. Does not ferment lactose 8. Facultative anaerobe	3. Siderophore	5. Diarrhea – only fluid and electrolyte replacement is required

4. Salmonella typhi

Salmonella typhi is an exception in that it is **not zoonotic** (i.e. an infectious disease that is carried by animals and that can be transmitted and infect humans), and instead, is carried solely by humans. Infection with *Salmonella typhi*, which is a facultative intracellular paraside, occurs via fecal-oral transmission. Infection with *Salmonella typhi* can cause typhoid fever, whose symptoms often resemble those found in patients with appendicitis. Some individuals recovering from typhoid fever become chronic carriers. These individuals, who are asymptomatic and not actively infected, continue to carry *Salmonella typhi* in their gallbladders and excrete the bacterium constantly.

Clinical Manifestations	Diagnostics	Virulence Factors	Treatment
SALMONELLA TYPHI **(non-thyphi groups of Salmonella; not zoonotic)**			
1. Typhoid fever, also called enteric fever. Symptoms include fever, abdominal pain (either diffuse or located in the right lower quadrant), hepatosplenomega ly **and rose spots on abdomen; a light rash that consists of small pink marks visible only on light-skinned**	**Gram stain:** 1. Gram (-) rods **Culture:** 2. Urine, blood, CSF; EMB (Eosin methylene blue) / MacConke	1. Flagella (H antigen) – motile 2. Capsule (Vi antigen): protects against intracellula r killing 3. Siderophor e	1. Ciprofloxacin 2. Ceftriaxone 3. Trimethoprim & Sulfamethoxazo le 4. Azithromycin

people.	y agar		
2. Chronic carrier state	3. Produces H2S		
	Metabolism:		
	4. Catalase (+)		
	5. Oxidase (-)		
	6. Ferments glucose		
	7. Does not ferment lactose		
	8. Facultative anaerobe		

SHIGELLA

There are four species of *Shigella*, which incude *Shigella dysenteriae*, *Shigella flexneri*, *Shigella boydii* and *Shigella sonnei*; all of which are non-motile. *Shigella* does not produce H2S, nor does it ferment lactose – both of which are distinguishing factors allowing differentiation of *Shigella* from *Escherichia coli*, which is a lactose fermenter, and *Salmonella*, which is a lactose fermenter as well as a H2S producer. Shigella, which is always pathogenic, is never considered part of the natural intestinal flora.

5. Shigella dysenteriae

Infection with *Shigella dysenteriae*, which is harbored solely by humans, occurs via fecal-oral transmission. *Shigella dysenteriae* is a species of the rod-shaped *Shigella*, which are Gram-negative, non-motile, non-spore-forming and faculatively anaerobic.

Clinical Manifestations	Diagnostics	Virulence Factors	Treatment
SHIGELLA DYSENTERIAE			
1. Shiga toxin: inactivates the 60S ribosome, inhibiting protein synthesis and killing intestinal cells **Symptoms include bloody**	**Gram stain:** 1. Gram (-) rods **Culture:** 2. Stool (never part of the normal	1. Non-motile (no H antigen) 2. Invades submucosa of the intestinal tract, but not the lamina	1. Fluoroquinolones 2. Trimethoprim and sulfamethoxazole IgA is best for immunity

| diarrhea with mucus and pus – resembles *E. coli* | intestinal flora); EMB (Eosin methylene blue) / MacConkey agar

3. Does not produce H2S

Metabolism:

4. Catalase (+)

5. Oxidase (-)

6. Ferments glucose

7. Does not ferment lactose

8. Facultative anaerobe | propria | |

VIBRIONACEAE

1. **Vibrio cholera**

Vibrio cholera, which is transmitted via the fecal-oral transmission route, is a short, curved, comma-shaped Gram-negative rod with a single (H antigen) polar flagellum. Typically contracted through contaminated water, *Vibrio cholera* can cause cholera – a diarrheal disease. Recent epidemics have arisen in Latin American countries in 1991 and in Bangladesh in 1993, after monsoon floods lead to the contamination of water. Once infected, *Vibrio cholera* bacteria attach to the epithelial cells and release the cholera toxin choleragen. Cholera, which is accompanied with the sudden onset of watery diarrhea (rice water stools), can cause death by dehydration. In extreme cases, one liter of fluid is lost per hour.

Clinical Manifestations	Diagnostics	Virulence Factors	Treatment
VIBRIO CHOLERA			
1. Choleragen (enterotoxin): like LT of *E. coli*, *Vibrio Cholera* increases cAMP, causing secretion of electrolytes from the intestinal epithelium. This leads to	**Gram Stain:** 1. Short, curved, comma-shaped, gram (-) rods with a single polar flagellum **Culture:**	1. Flagellum (H antigen) – motile 2. Mucinase: digests mucous layer, allowing *Vibrio Cholera* to attach to	1. Replace fluids 2. Doxycycline 3. Fluoroquinolone

| the secretion of fluid into the intestinal tract

Cholera, which causes death by dehydration, is characterized by severe diarrhea with rice water stools. | TCBS agar

2. Flat yellow colonies

3. Dark field microscopy of

stool

- motile organisms

immobilized with

antiserum

Metabolism:

4. Ferments sugar

(except lactose) | cells

3. Fimbriae: helps with attachment

to cells

4. Non-invasive | |

2. Campylobacter jejuni

Campylobacter jejuni – a curved, Gram-negative rod with a single polar flagellum, is similar in appearance to *Vibrio Cholera,* and is one of the three leading causes of diarrhea in the world. Like most *Salmonella, Campylobacter jejuni* is also zoonotic and encountered in wild and domestic animals and poultry. The bacterium is most commonly transmitted via the fecal-oral route, through contaminated water or unpasteurized milk. Upon entry into the body, the bacterium colonizes the lining of the small intestine and spread systematically. An active *Campylobacter jejuni* excretes an LT toxin as well as an unknown cytotoxic that destroys mucosal cells. Once infected, an individual with the disease will experience headaches, as well as develop a fever – both of which are early symptoms indicating onset of an illness – followed by bloody loose diarrhea and abdominal days half a day later.

Clinical Manifestations	Diagnostics	Virulence Factors	Treatment
CAMPYLOBACTER JEJUNI			
1. Enterotoxin: Similar to cholera toxin and LT of *E. coli* **2. Cytotoxin: Destroys mucosal cells** **Other symptoms include secretory or bloody**	**Gram Stain:** 1. Curved Gram (-) rods with a single polar flagellum **Culture:** Stool; EMB (Eosin methylene blue) / MacConkey	1. Flagella (H antigen) – motile 2. Invasiveness	1. Fluoroquinolone 2. Erythromycin 3. Ciprofloxacin

diarrhea	agar		
(– this is associated with Guillain-Barre syndrome, acute	2. Optimum temperature is 42°C		
neuromuscular paralysis; autoimmune)	**Metabolism:** 3. Oxidase (+) 4. Does not ferment lactose 5. Microphilic aerobe		

3. Helicobacter pylori –

Helicobacter pylori is the leading cause of duodenal ulcers and chronic gastritis (i.e. inflammation of the stomach). Besides this, it is also the second leading cause of gastric ulcers (stomach ulcers), second only to aspirin products.

Clinical Manifestations	Diagnostics	Virulence Factors	Treatment

1. Duodenal ulcers	Gram stain:		1. Bismuth, ampicillin,
2. Chronic gastritis	1. Curved gram (-) rods with a tuft of polar flagellum		metronidazole and tetracycline
	Metabolism:		2. Clarithromycin and omeprazole
	2. Urease (+)		
	3. Microaerobe (microaerophilic)		– Both these treatments reduce duodenal ulcer relapse

PSEUDOMONADACEAE

Pseudomonas can cause pneumonia and sepsis. But treatment of Pseudomonas is often, due to their antibiotic-resistant properties, challenging and often necessitates the provision of two antibiotics with anti-pseudomonal activity.

1. Pseudomonas aeruginosa

Pseudomonas aeruginosa – a Gram-negative, non-lactose-fermenting, obligate aerobic rod – is significant for two reasons:

not only does it colonize and infect hospitalized patients that are sick and immunocompromised, but it is also resistant to essential every antibiotic. *Pseudomonas aeruginosa* produces two pigments: a green fluorescent pigment called **pyoverdin** and a blue pigment called **pyocyanin**. These two pigments are what colors colonies and infected wound dressings green-bluish. The hospital-acquired Gram-negative organism however, has weak invasive ability and is thus rare to infect healthy individuals. It is therefore said to be an 'opportunistic' organism.

Clinical Manifestations	Diagnostics	Virulence Factors	Treatment
PSEUDOMONAS AERUGINOSA			

| Pseudomonas exotoxin A inhibits protein synthesis by blocking EF2 (Elongation Factor 2) – same mechanisms as employed by the diphtheria toxin

1. Pneumonia (cystic fibrosis and in immunosuppressed patients)
2. Osteomyelitis (in diabetics, IV drug users and in children)
3. Burn wound infections
4. Sepsis
5. Urinary tract infection
6. Endocarditis (in IV drug users)
7. Malignant external otitis
8. Corneal infections in contact lens wearers | **Gram Stain:**

1. Gram (-) rods

Culture:
Blood agar

2. Greenish-metallic

with a fruit smell

Metabolism:
3. Oxidase (+)
4. Does not ferment lactose

5. Obligate aerobe | 1. Polar flagellum (H antigen) – motile
2. Hemolysin
3. Collagenase
4. Elastase
5. Fibrinolysin
6. Phospholipase C
7. DNAase
8. Antiphagocytic capsule (some strains) | 1. Ticarcillin
2. Timentin
3. Carbenicillin
4. Piperacillin
5. Mezlocillin
6. Ciprofloxacin
7. Imipenem
8. Tobramycin
9. Aztreonam |

BACTEROIDACEAE

In humans, 99% of the normal flora of the intestinal tract is composed of obligate anerobi Gram-negative rods, which include the family Bacteroidaceae. Organisms belonging to this family are also found in the vagina and in the mouth.

1. Bacteroides fragilis

Bacteroides fragilis, which is part of the normal flora of the intestine, is a Gram-negative, anaerobic rod that does not contain lipid A and thus has no endotoxins. Despite its low virulence, the bacteria can cause an infection once it enters into the peritoneal cavity. Inside the cavity, the organism causes the formation of abscesses, which is often accompanied by fever and systematic spread.

Clinical Manifestations	Diagnostics	Virulence Factors	Treatment
BACTEROIDES FRAGILIS			

| 1. Does not contain Lipid A – Abscesses in gastrointestinal tract, pelvis and in the lungs | Gram Stain: 1. Gram (-) rods 2. Non-spore forming c 3. Polysaccharide capsule Metabolism: 4. Anaerobe | Infection occurs once *Bacteroides fragilis* enters the peritoneal cavity | 1. Metronidazole 2. Clindamycin 3. Chloramphenicol 4. Surgically drain abscess |

III. Gram-Negative Rods Related to Respiratory Tract Infections

Haemophilus infiuenzae, Bordetella pertussis and *Legionella pneumophila* are all Gram-negative rods that are grouped together due to the fact that they are acquired through the respiratory tract.

Haemophilus

Haemophilus means 'blood-loving.' Organisms belonging to this family thus require blood for growth. In other words, they can only develop in a medium that contains blood.

1. Haemophilus influenzae

Haemophilus infiuenzae is an obligate parasite present in humans that is transmitted via the respiratory route. It requires two factors for growth (both of which are found in blood): The X factor, that is Hematin, and the V factor: NAD+. The organism comprises a capsule – of which there are six types: a, b, c, d, e and f – they are capable of conferring virulence. Of these capsules, type b is considered to be the most invasive one, and the leading cause of *Haemophilus infiuenzae* disease in children, which includes meningitis, acute epiglottis and septic arthritis. At the same time, non-encapsulated strains of *Haemophilus infiuenzae,* which are referred to as non-typeable, can also colonise the upper respiratory tract in children and adults. These non-typeable strains however, lack virulent invasiveness and only lead to local infections. In children, they often cause otitis media and in adults, in the presence of another pre-existing lung disease, they are responsible for other diseases affecting respiratory function.

Clinical Manifestations	Diagnostics	Virulence Factors	Treatment
HAEMOPHILUS INFLUENZA			

| I. Encapsulated *Haemophilus infiuenzae*:
 1. Meningitis (*Haemophilus infiuenzae* **type b is the primary cause of meningitis in infants age 3 – 36 months); can lead to complications that include retardation, seizures, deafness, and death**
 2. Acute epiglottis
 3. Septic arthritis in infants
 4. Sepsis, especially in patients without functioning spleens 5. Pneumonia

 II. Non – encapsulated *Haemophilus* | **Gram Stain:**
 1. Gram (-) rods

 Culture:
 Blood agar that has been heated to 80 °C for 15 min – this is now called **chocolate agar**
 2. The organism grows best when the chocolate agar is placed in an environment high in CO2 (at 37 °C)
 3. Fluorescent antibodies (ELiSA and latex particle agglutination)
 4. Positive Quellung test (because of its capsule) | 1. Capsule: there are 6 types a - f, of which type b is the most virulent
 2. Attachment pili (FHA)
 3. IgA1 protease | **1. Second or third generation cephalosporins** – this is because *Haemophilus infiuenzae* can become ampicillin resistant by plasmids

 2. Hib vaccines: DTaP and oral polio are given at the same time – in the US, this has drastically reduced the incidence of Hib infection (meningitis, acute epiglottis, etc.)

 3. Passive immunization: In order to increase passive antibody transfer |

infiuenzae:			(through breast
1. Otitis media			milk) and
2. Sinusitis			transfer of
3. COPD			immunity,
exacerbation			mothers are
and			immunized
pneumonia			during the 8th
			month of the
			pregnancy

2. Haemophilus ducreyi (STD)

Haemophilus ducreyi causes chancroid, a sexually transmitted disease. Infected patients will experience a painful genital ulcer, as well as painful unilateral swollen inguinal lymph nodes that are pus-releasing after becoming matted and rupturing.

Clinical Manifestations	Diagnostics	Virulence Factors	Treatment

HAEMOPHILUS DUCREYI

1. Chancroid: Painful genital ulcer, typically associated with unilateral swollen lymph nodes that rupture and release pus	Gram Stain: 1. Gram (-) rods Culture: 2. Ulcer exudates and pus from lymph node	1. No capsule	1. Azithromycin or erythromycin 2. Ceftriaxone 3. Ciprofloxacin

Bordetella

3. Bordetella pertussis

Bordetella pertussis is a highly contagious disease, transmitted via the respiratory route, which causes a whooping cough. The organism is, because of its virulence factors, capable of attaching itself to the ciliated epithelial cells of the trachea and the bronchi, which it then destroys, causing a whooping cough. Demographics that belong to the high-risk groups include infants age one and younger and adults as vaccine-acquired immunity wears off.

Clinical Manifestations	Diagnostics	Virulence Factors	Treatment
BORDETELLA PERTUSSIS			
Whooping cough **1. Catarrhal phase: (1 – 2 weeks); patient is high contagious – Symptoms include low-grade fever, a runny nose and a mild cough – During this stage: antibiotic susceptible 2. Paroxymal phase: (2 – 10 weeks); – Whoop = bursts of non-productive coughs – Increased number of**	Graim stain: 1. Gram (-) rod Culture: 2. Bordet-Gengou media: potatoes, blood and glycerol agar with penicillin added 3. Serologic tests (ELISA): collect a specimen from the posterior pharynx on a calcium alginate swab as *Bordetella pertussis* does not grow on cotton 4. For rapid	1. Pertussis toxin: The toxin activates G proteins that increase cAMP, resulting in – Increased histamine sensitivity, – Increased insulin release, and – Increased lymphocytes in blood 2. Extra-cytoplasmic adenylate cyclase: "weakens" neutrophils lymphocytes, and	1. **Erythromycin** (most effective when given before the paroxymal stage, i.e. during the catarrhal phase) 2. Vaccine: D(a)PT, – Diptheria, acellular Pertussis and Tetanus (vaccine may cause rash and fever, rarely systemic disease); often given to

lymphocytes in blood smear – During this stage, antibiotics are ineffective 3. Convalescent phase	diagnosis: direct flourescein-labeled antibodies applied to nasopharyngeal specimens 5. PCR detection of bacterial DNA in respiratory secretions	monocytes 3. Filamentous hemagglutinin (FHA): This is a pili rod that extends from the surface of the organism, allowing it to bind to the ciliated epithelial cells of the bronchi 4. Tracheal cytotoxin: Kills ciliated epithelial cells	patients age 2, 4, 6 and 16 months and children between the age of 4 and 6 3. Use erythromycin to treat household contacts

Legionella

4. Legionella pneumophila

Legionella pneumophila, an aerobic Gram-negative rod, is ubiquitous in both manmade and natural water environments. Infection occurs following inhalation of aerosolized contaminated water. Other sources that have led to outbreaks of the bacterium include air conditioners, whirlpools, and cooling towers. Upon entry into the body, the facultative intracellular parasite colonizes the lower respiratory tract where it is enveloped by macrophages. Following phagocytosis, the organism inhibits phagosome-lysosome function, all whilst continuing to grow within the cell/s. *Legionella pneumophila* can cause a variety of diseases, ranging from Pontiac fever (a flulike, asymptomatic infection) to severe pneumonia that is also referred to as Legionnaires' disease (characterized by high fevers and severe pneumonia).

Clinical Manifestations	Diagnostics	Virulence Factors	Treatment
LEGIONELLA PNEUMOPHILA			
1. Cytotoxin: **Kills hamster ovary cells** **2. Pontiac fever:** **Symptoms include headache, fever, fatigue and myalgia; self-limiting but recovery typically occurs within**	**Gram Stain:** 1. Gram (-) rod (faint) **Culture:** 2. Buffered charcoal yeast extract agar (of which L-cysteine is a critical ingredient) 3. Serologic tests (IFA and ELISA) 4. Urinary antigen	1. Facultative intracellular parasite 2. Cu-Zn superoxide dismutase and catalase-peroxidase – this protects the bacteria from macrophage superoxide and	1. Azithromycin 2. Levofloxacin 3. Doxycycline

a week 3. **Legionnaires' Disease: Symptoms include atypical pneumonia high fevers, non-productive cough**	can be detected by radioimmunoassay; high sensitivity and specificity will remain (+) for months after infection – urine antigen test can only detect *Legionella pneumophila* **serogroup 1**, but this makes up 90% of cases 5. Facultative intracellular parasite (inside alveolar macrophages) 6. Individuals with comprised immune systems are particularly susceptible	hydrogen peroxide oxidative burst 3. Pili and flagella – these promote attachment and invasion of host cell 4. Secretion of protein toxins 102 like RNAase, phospholipase A and phospholipase C	

IV. Gram-Negative Obligate Intracellular Parasites

Chlamydia, Rickettsia and *Ehrlicihia* are groups of Gram-negative obligate intracellular parasites. For survival, these bacteria groups must reside within animal cells, as they require ATP from their host for their cellular activity. Because of this, these bacteria are sometimes referred to as **energy parasites**. Both *Chlamydia* and *Rickettsia* use ATP – ADP translocators, the difference being that while *Rickettsia* can oxidize certain molecules and form ATP through oxidative phosphorylation, *Chlamydia* has no available mechanism for ATP synthesis. All three bacterial groups cause an array of different human diseases. While *Chlamydia* spreads by person-to-person contact however, *Rickettsia* is transmitted by an arthropod vector.

CHLAMYDIA

Chlamydia are very small Gram-negative bacteria and differentiates itself from the other Gram-negative bacteria by the fact that it lacks a peptidoglycan layer and has no muramic acid. Chlamydia, which are obligate intracellular parasites that steal ATP from its host with ATP-ADP translocator, are responsible for causing a variety of diseases, including conjunctivitis, cervicitis and pneumonia.

1. Chlamydia trachomatis

Chlamydia trachomatis is a disease affecting humans that is transmitted via direct contact. Chlamydia trachomatis primarily causes infection in the eyes, lungs and the genitals and is also responsible for trachoma; a type of chronic conjunctivitis that is the most common cause of preventable blindness in the world. Trachoma (caused by Chlamydia trachomatis serotypes A, B and C), which develops gradually over a period of 10 – 15 years, is classified as a 'disease of poverty,' affecting primarily poorer areas and countries where hygiene is poor. The disease spreads via hand-to-hand transmission of infected eye secretions, direct personal contact, and by sharing clothes and towels that have been contaminated.

Clinical Manifestations	Diagnostics	Virulence Factors	Treatment
CHLAMYDIA TRACHOMATIS			
1. Serotypes A, B, C: **– Trachoma: causes scarring of the inside of the eyelid, which results in the redirection of the eyelashes onto the corneal surface (This, over time, results in corneal scarring and blindness)** **2. Serotypes D-K:** **– Inclusion**	**Gram Stain:** 1. Gram (-), but lacks peptidoglycan layer and muramic acid **Culture:** Cannot be grown on artificial media. *Chlamydia* is thus most commonly cultured in certain cell lines, e.g. McCoy cells 2. Conjunctiva surface – for	1. Resistant to lysozyme (because their cell walls lack muramic acid) 2. Prevents phagosome-lysosome fusion 3. Non-motile 4. No pili 5. No exotoxins	For genital and eye infections: 1. Doxycycline (only for adults) 2. Erythromycin (especially for infants and pregnant women) 3. Azithromycin

conjunctivitis (opthalmia neonatorum) – Infant pneumonia – Urethritis, cervicitis, and PID (pelvic inflammatory disease) in women – Nongonoccal urethritis, epididymitis, prostatitis in men *Complications of chlamydial genital tract infections:* – Sterility, ectopic pregnancy, and chronic pain may occur after PID – Reiter's syndrome, tried of conjunctivitis, urethritis and arthritis – Perihepatitis (Fitz-Hugh-Curtis	inclusion conjunctivitis (ophthalmia neonatorum), scrapings from the surface of the conjunctiva will exhibit intracytolasmic inclusion bodies within the conjunctival epithelial cells (which will contain glycogen and thus stain with iodine or giemsa) 3. Genital secretions will not show any gram (-) diplococci 4. Urethritis is most commonly diagnosed by polymerase chain reaction of urethral swab or urine sample 5. Immuno-fluorescent slide test: infected genital or ocular secretions are		For any chlamydial eye infection, **systemic treatment** is required – this is particularly important for infants that can develop pneumonia following chlamydial conjunctivit is

Syndrome) **3. Serotypes L1, L2 and L3 :** **-** **Lymphogranulo ma venereum**	placed on a slide and stained with fluorescein-conjugated anti-chlamydial antibodies 6. Serologies: requires examination of blood for elevated titers of anti-chlamydial antibodies with complement fixation and immunofluoresce nce tests 7 Lymphogranulom a venereum: serologic tests, Frei test (rarely used) **Metabolism (cell cycle):** 1. Elementary body dense spherule that infects cells 2. Initial body:		

	After Elementary body enters the cell, it it transformed into an initial body – that is larger and osmotically fragile – that can reproduce (binary fission) – that requires ATP from host cell(s) – the initial body is then transformed back into the elementary body, leaving the cell to infect other cells	

2. **Chlamydia pneumoniae**

Chlamydia pneumoniae, transmitted via the respiratory route from human to human, is a strain TWAR (Taiwan acute respiratory agent); a small Gram-negative bacterium with a complex cell cycle that resembles that of Chlamydia trachomatis. Typically acquired from a healthy person, *Chlamydia pneumoniae* is a form of community-acquired pneumonia that is characterized as being 'atypical'.

Clinical Manifestations	Diagnostics	Virulence Factors	Treatment
	CHLAMYDIA PNEUMONIAE		
1. Atypical pneumonia : **Viral-like atypical pneumonia, with fever and dry and a non-productive cough in young adults –** similar to *Mycoplasma pneumonia*	**Gram Stain:** 1. Gram (-), lacks peptidoglycan layer **Culture:** 2. Conjunctiva surface, genital secretions) 3. No gram (-) diplococci 4. Immuno-fluorescent slide test 5. Serologies – requires examination of the blood for elevated titers of antibodies with complement fixation and immune-	Cell cycle similar to above (to *Chlamydia trachomatis*) – must infect another cell to reproduce	1. Doxycycline 2. Erythromycin

| | fluorescence tests

6.
Intracytoplasmic inclusion bodies do not stain with iodine | | |
|---|---|---|---|

RICKETTSIA

Rickettsia is a non-motile, Gram-negative rod/coccoid-shaped bacterium that shares many of the characteristics of Chlamydia. Like Chlamydia, Rickettsiae are small in size and are obligate intracellular parasites (i.e. they cannot make their own ATP) that steal ATP from host cells. There are, however, also many differences between the two: Rickettsia, for example, requires an arthropod vector (except for Q fever). Furthermore, Rickettsia can replicate freely within the cytoplasm – whereas Chlamydia replicates in endosomes. While Chlamydia damages columnar epithelium – Rickettsia damages endothelial cells that line blood vessels. Lastly, Rickettsia causes different illnesses, including headaches, high fevers and rashes.

1. **Rickettsia rickettsii**

Rickettsia rickettsia, transmitted by dog and wood ticks, is a Gram-negative, coccobacillus, intracellular bacterium that causes Rocky

Mountain spotted fever. The disease – which becomes visible roughly one week after a person is bitten by the dog tick *Dermacentor variabilis* (in Eastern US) or by the wood tick *Dermacentor andersoni* (in Western US) – is characterized by fever, bad headaches, conjunctival redness and a rash that appears on the wrists, palms, ankles and soles at first instance, before spreading to the trunk. Because the tick only transmits the bacterium during 6 - 10 hours of feeding, early discovery and removal of ticks can prevent infection. Rocky Mountain spotted fever is most widespread across the southeastern tick belt of the US, although cases have been reported in almost every state. While the disease typically only lasts three weeks, it can be fatal in some cases – particularly where antibiotic therapy is delayed.

Clinical Manifestations	Diagnostics	Virulence Factors	Treatment
RICKETTSIA RICKETTSIA			
1. Rocky Mountain Spotted Fever: Symptoms include the following: **– Fever** **– Conjunctival injection (redness)** **– Severe**	1. Clinical exam 2. ELISA (direct immuno-fluorescent exam) of skin biopsy from rash site 3. Serology 4. Positive		1. Doxycycline 2. Chloramphenicol

headaches – Rash on wrists, palms, ankles and soles (at first), which becomes more generalized and centrifugal (at a later stage)	(+) Weil-Felix reaction: – Positive: OX-2 – Positive: OX-19		

2. Rickettsia akari

Rickettsia akari, which is transmitted by mites on house mice (i.e. mites that live on the house mice), causes **rickettsialpox** – a mild, self-limiting, zoonotic, febrile illness. Early symptoms include localized red skin bumps (papules) near the mite bite, that later develop into a blister (vesicle), before progressing into a fever and headache a few days later, at which point other vesicles will appear all over the body.

Clinical Manifestations	Diagnostics	Virulence Factors	Treatment
RICKETTSIA AKARI			

1. Rickettsial Pox: – Vesicular rash that resembles chicken pox – Typically resolves over 2 weeks	1. Clinical exam 2. Negative (-) Weil-Felix reaction		1. Doxycycline 2. Chloramphenicol

EHRLICIHIA

1. Ehrlichia canis/chaffeensis

The organism *Ehrlichia chaffeensis* (Human Monocytic Ehrlichiosis) – an obligate intracellular Gram-negative organism – is responsible for Ehrlichiosis; a tick-borne disease that is similar to Rocky Mountain spotted fever without a rash. The disease spreads through tick infection and arises particularly in the mid-Atlantic, southern, south-central regions of the US.

Clinical Manifestations	Diagnostics	Virulence Factors	Treatment
EHRLICHIA CHAFFEENSIS			

1. Human Ehrlichiosis: **– Similar to Rocky Mountain spotted Fever** **– But a rash is rare**	1. Rise in acute and convalescent antibody titers 2. Ehrlichial inclusion bodies (morula bodies) are sometimes seen in leukocytes on blood smears 3. PCR testing		1. Doxycycline 2. Rifampin (resistant to chloramphenicol)

V. Gram-Negative SPIROCHETES

Spirochetes are Gram-negative, spiral-shaped organisms that are extremely small in size (they are too small to be seen using light microscope). They are tightly coiled, spin around and have specialized axial flagella, **periplasmic flagella**, which run sideways along the spirochete. Like other Gram-negative bacteria, spirochetes contain a thin peptidoglycan cell wall that is surrounded by LPS contained in the outer lipoprotein membrane. Despite being a small group of bacteria, they can be seriously pathogenic for humans, causing diseases such as Lyme disease, yaws, syphilis, and relapsing fever. Spirochetes replicate by transverse fission and require special procedures to be seen, such as immunofluorescence, dark field microscopy and silver stains.

TREPONEMA

Treponemes do not produce any toxins or any tissue-destroying enzymes. Instead, the diseases caused by this group of organisms result from the immune responses of its host, such as granuloma formation, inflammatory cell infiltrates, and proliferative vascular changes.

1. Treponema pallidum

Treponema pallidum is an infectious organism that causes syphilis, a sexually transmitted disease. The agent enters the body by penetrating intact mucous membranes or by passing through epithelial abrasions. Infection can also occur through skin contact with a Treponema pallidum infected ulcer. As soon as the infection occurs, the spirochetes begin disseminating throughout the body. An untreated infection will progress through three clinical stages, including a latent period between the secondary and the tertiary stage.

Clinical Manifestations	Diagnostics	Virulence Factors	Treatment
TREPONEMA PALLIDUM			

1. Syphilis – Primary stage: Painless ulcer (chancre) **– Secondary stage: Symptoms include a rash on palms and soles; – (condyloma laturn) painless wart-like lesion in moist areas, e.g. vulva and the scrotum; – the central nervous system, eyes, bones, kidneys, or joints may be involved – Latent stage (latent syphilis): 25% may relapse back to the secondary stage and develop secondary**	**1. Dark field microscopy** (to examine cutaneous Q lesions) Morphology: Gram (-), thick rigid spirals **2. ELISA or silver stain** **3. Non-specific treponemal test** (VDRL; RPR) **4. Specific treponemal test** (FTA-ABS; MHA-TP) – pregnant women must all be screened with VDRL because antibiotic treatment before four months of gestation prevents congenital syphilis	1. Motile: Six axial filaments wind around *Treponema pallidum* between the peptidoglycan layer and the outer cell membrane (contraction of these leads to spinning motion)	1. Penicillin G 2. Erythromycin 3. Doxycycline Jarisch - Herxheimer reaction: acute worsening of symptoms after antibiotics are started

stage symptoms again – **Tertiary stage: (33%):** **Symptoms** **include** **gummas of** **skin and bone,** **–** **cardiovascular** **syphilis** **(aortic** **aneurysm), –** **neurosyphilis** **(may get the** **Argyll-** **Robertson** **pupil)** **– Congenital:** **Contracted in-** **utero, occurs** **in the fetus of** **an infected** **women.** **Fetuses with** **an infection** **have a high** **mortality rate** **and almost all** **that survive** **will develop** **early or late** **congenital**	5. PCR detection (polymerase chain reaction) of bacterial DNA 6. **Microaerophilic** **, very sensitive** **to high** **temperatures**		

syphilis.			

BORRELIA

Bacterial species belonging to the spirochete class of the genus *Borrelia* are corkscrew-shaped and larger in size compared to the *Treponema* species. They can be observed using a light microscope with Wright or Giemsa stains. Borrelia causes a variety of diseases, ranging from relapsing fever to Lyme disease; both of which are transmitted via insect vectors.

1. Borrelia burgdorferi

Borrelia burgdorferi is the bacterial species responsible for Lyme disease. They are transmitted via Ixodes ticks from white-footed mice and white-tailed deer (*Ixodes scapularis* in the East and the Midwest and *Ixodes pacificus* on the West coast). Lyme disease, which in many ways resembles syphilis, is not sexually transmitted, although both diseases are caused by spirochetes. Like syphilis, Lyme disease also occurs in three stages – consisting of an early localized stage, an early disseminated stage and a late stage – and can also cause chronic problems years after the infection (late stage Lyme disease and tertiary syphilis).

Clinical Manifestations	Diagnostics	Virulence Factors	Treatment
BORRELIA BURGDORFERI			
1. Lyme Disease – Early localized stage (stage 1): Erythema chronicum migrans (ECM) **– Early disseminated (stage 2): Multiple smaller ECMs, –**	1. Clinical observation 2. Elevated levels of antibodies against *Borrelia burgdorferi* can detected by ELISA 3. Western immunoblot		1. Doxycycline (acute) 2. Amoxicillin (acute) 3. Ceftriaxone for neurologic disease

| (neurologic) aseptic meningitis, cranial palsies (called Bell's palsy) and peripheral neuropathy, – (cardiac) transient heart block or myocariditis, – (knee) brief arthritis attacks of large joints

– Late stage (stage 3): Chronic arthritis, encephalopathy | 4. Microaerophilic | | 4. Penicillin G (chronic) |

2. Borrelia recurrentis

In total, there are 18 different Borrelia species that can cause relapsing fever, but only one of these – *Borrelia recurrentis* – is transmitted to humans via the body louse (*Pediculus humanus*), with all other ones being transmitted to humans via the *Ornithodoros* tick. Relapsing fever is an infectious bacterial disease characterized by recurring episodes of fever. Once Borrelia recurrentis has been transmitted, it disseminates via the blood, causing a high fever that is accompanied by headaches, muscle aches and chills. As the illness progresses, rash and meningeal involvement can follow. After 3 - 6 days, drenching sweats, fever and symptoms may resolve and the patient remains afebrile (i.e. not feverish) for around 8 days, but then relapses for another 3 - 6 days. These relapses continue, although they will become increasingly shorter as the afebrile intervals become increasingly longer.

Clinical Manifestations	Diagnostics	Virulence Factors	Treatment
BORRELIA RECURRENTIS			
1. Relapsing fever **– Recurring fever about every 8 days.** **– Fever breaks with drenching sweats.** **– Rash and splenomegaly.** **– Occasional meningeal involvement.**	1. During febrile periods: Dark field microscopy of blood drawn during febrile periods and blood culture from febrile periods. 3. Wright's or Giemsa stain – stained peripheral blood smears show organisms (70% of the time)	1. Antigenic variation of outer membrane **Vmp lipoproteins** allow the bacterium to escape phagocytosis and opsonization 2. No toxins	1. Doxycycline 2. Erythromycin 3. Penicillin G

	4. Serologies 5. Microaerophilic		

3. Borrelia hermsii

Borrelia hermsii is a rodent-associated spirochete bacterium that is the primary and most common cause of tick-borne relapsing fever in North America. It is transmitted through the bite of the soft-bodied tick *Ornithodoros hermsi*.

Clinical Manifestations	Diagnostics	Virulence Factors	Treatment
	BORRELIA HERMSII		

1. Relapsing fever **– Recurring fever about every 8 days** **– Fever breaks with drenching sweats** **– Rash and splenomegaly** **– Occasional meningeal involvement**	1. During febrile periods: Dark field microscopy of blood drawn during febrile periods and blood culture from febrile periods 3. Wright's or Giemsa stain – stained peripheral blood smears show organisms (70% of the time) 4. Serologies 5. Microaerophilic	1. Antigenic variation of outer membrane **Vmp lipoproteins** allow the bacterium to escape phagocytosis and opsonization 2. No toxins	1. Doxycycline 2. Erythromycin 3. Penicillin G

Dr. Joshua Larsen

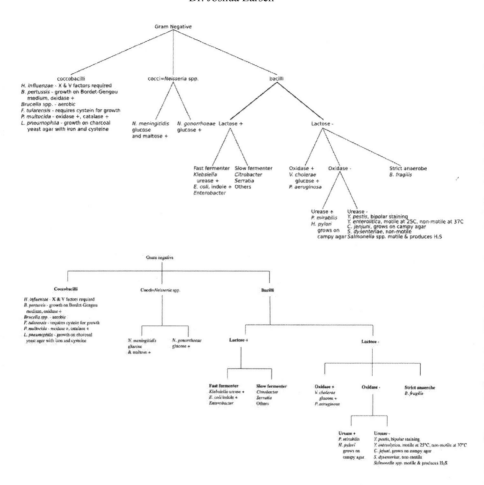

Gram Negative

coccobacilli
- *H. influenzae* - X & V factors required
- *B. pertussis* - growth on Bordet-Gengou medium, oxidase +
- *Brucella* spp. - aerobic
- *F. tularensis* - requires cystein for growth
- *P. multocida* - oxidase +, catalase +
- *L. pneumophila* - growth on charcoal yeast agar with iron and cysteine

cocci=*Neisseria* spp.

N. meningitidis glucose and maltose +

N. gonorrhoeae glucose +

bacilli

Lactose +
- Fast fermenter
  Klebsiella urease +
  E. coli, indole +
  Enterobacter
- Slow fermenter
  Citrobacter
  Serratia
  Others

Lactose -
- Oxidase +
  V. cholerae glucose +
  P. aeruginosa
- Oxidase -
  - Urease +
    P. mirabilis
    H. pylori grows on campy agar
  - Urease -
    Y. pestis, bipolar staining
    Y. enterolitica, motile at 25C, non-motile at 37C
    C. jejuni, grows on campy agar
    S. dysenteriae, non-motile
    Salmonella spp. motile & produces H₂S
- Strict anaerobe
  B. fragilis

6. MISCELLANEOUS BACTERIA

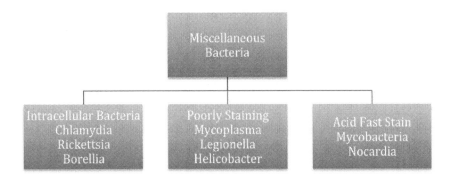

<u>ACTINOMYCETES</u>

Actinomycetes are bacteria that act like fungi. There are two clinically significant actinomycetes that cause human disease - *Actinomyces israelli* and *Nocardia,* both of which are Gram-positive rods that will be discussed in this section.

1. Actinomyces israelli

Actinomyces israelli, found in the normal natural flora of the mouth and the GI tract, is a beaded, filamentous anaerobic prokaryotic organism that can cause eroding abscesses, which are followed by trauma to mucous membranes of the mouth or GI tract. Depending of the site of infection, the infection is referred to as oral cervicofacial actinomycosis (where the infection develops inside the neck, jaw or mouth), abdominal actinomycosis (where the infection develops inside the abdomen), or thoracic actinomycosis (where the infection develops inside the lungs and/or associated airways).

Clinical Manifestations	Diagnostics	Virulence Factors	Treatment
ACTINOMYCES ISRAELLI			
1. Actinomycosis **- Abscess with draining sinuses** **- Initial lesion involves face and neck (rest chest and abdomen)** **- Not communicable**	**Gram Stain:** 1. Gram (+), long branching filaments **Culture:** 2. Hard, yellow granules (sulfur granules) formed in pus 3. Culture of pus or tissue **Metabolism:**		1. Prolonged penicillin G and surgical drainage

	4. Anaerobe		
	5. Immune-fluorescence		

2. Nocardia asteroids

Nocardia asteroids, typically found in soil, forms weak (poorly staining) Gram-positive, and partly acid-fast beaded branching thin filaments. Individuals taking steroids are at a particular list of contracting the bacterium. Nocardia infections are routinely misdiagnosed as tuberculosis because of its acid-fast properties and because it has the same disease process. Nocardia, like tuberculosis, enters the body through inhalation and grows in the lungs where it produces abscesses and cavities. A Nocardia infection can also lead to erosions in the pleural space and blood-bourne dissemination, the latter of which can result in abscesses in other organs including the brain.

Clinical Manifestations	Diagnostics	Virulence Factors	Treatment
NOCARDIA ASTEROIDS			
1. Nocardiosis **- Abscesses in brain and kidneys in**	**Gram Stain:** 1. Gram (+) filaments, acid fast		1. Trimethoprim-sulfamethoxazole 2. In some cases, surgical drainage

immunodeficient points			may be necessary
2. Neumonia	**Metabolism:** 2. Aerobic		
3. Not communicable			

MYCOPLASMA

Mycoplasmataceae are unique bacteria; the smallest free-living organisms that can self-replicate – that also lack a peptidoglycan cell wall. This makes the cell membrane their only protective layer, inside which sterols are found that help protect the cell organelles from the exterior environment.

3. Mycoplasma pneumoniae

Mycoplasma pneumonia, which can cause self-limited bronchitis and pneumonia, is a contagious respiratory infection that is also the principal cause of bacterial bronchitis and pneumonia in teenagers and young adults. The disease caused by the bacterium, mycoplasma pneumonia, causes regular epidemics as it can spread easily and rapidly through contact with respiratory fluids and droplets. Upon entry into the body, the bacterium can attach itself to lung tissue and multiply, developing a full infection.

Clinical Manifestations	Diagnostics	Virulence Factors	Treatment
MYCOPLASMA PNEUMONIAE			
1. Atypical Pneumonia (also called *Walking pneumonia***)** **- Most common cause of pneumonia in teenagers and young adults** **- Symptoms include gradual development of a fever with a non-productive cough, sore throat and ear ache** **- Constitutional symptoms of fever,**	**Morphology:** 1. No cell wall 2. Bacterial membrane contains cholesterol 3. **Pleomorphic:** can appear rod-shaped with a pointed tip 4. Grown on artificial media, it requires lots of different lipids; characteristic of 'fried egg' colonies with	1. Produces hydrogen peroxide that damages respiratory tract cells 2. Antibodies against RBCs (cold agglutinins – an older test according to which, an antibody is produced in the blood that will cause RBCs to clump together when cooled during an active infection), brain, lung, and liver	1. Macrolide (Erythromycin, azithromycin) 2. Tetracycline (doxycycline) (penicillins and cephalosporins ineffective because no cell wall)

headache, malaise, and myalgias pronounced **- Minimal chest x-ray findings** **- Typically resolves spontaneously in 10-14 days**	a raised center 5. Serologies; cold-aglutinin titer (IgM autoAb's against type O blood cells) - non-specific **Metabolism:** 6. Facultative anaerobe 7. Requires cholesterol for membrane formation	cells produced during infection 3. Produces Community Acquired Respiratory Distress Syndrome (CARDS) toxin that leads to inflammation and airway dysfunction	

7. GENE REPLICATION AND GENETIC RECOMBINATION

Bacterial Gene Replication

The bacterial chromosome is composed of a double-stranded DNA molecule. Bacteria however, are haploid – i.e. they have a genome that consists of only a single DNA molecule.

Unlike eukaryotic cells, prokaryotes do not sexually reproduce with other bacteria, but instead undergo *gene replication*. During gene replication, an exact copy of their genome is produced.

Genetic Recombination

Bacteria have four ways in which they can exchange genetic fragments: transformation, conjugation, transduction and transposon or transposition. It is this exchange of genetic information that ensures survival – by increasing genetic diversity – and that allows the sharing of genes that code for proteins.

1. Transformation

Transformation is the intake or update of 'naked' DNA by **competent cells**, during which the DNA of a cell is altered as a result of the direct incorporation of exogenous genetic material (that is taken in through the cell membrane or membranes from the cell's surrounding). A 'state of competence' is a prerequisite for transformation to take place. Competence can occur naturally, as a response to the cell's environmental conditions, but can also be lab-induced. Within their environment, bacteria routinely encounter DNA and those bacterial cells capable of taking up foreign DNA are said to be competent. In other words, competence is the ability of a cell to incorporate DNA from its surroundings.

In competent bacterial cells, large molecules of DNA can pass through the cell wall and into the cytoplasm of that cell. At this point, **recombination** is necessary for the DNA to be incorporated into the **bacterial genome.** Transformation does not require cell-to-cell contact.

Bacterial transformation, as illustrated in the diagram below, occurs as follows:

1. **Step I:**
   - In the bacterial cell, DNA is found both in the cytoplasm (see number 1) and in the plasmid - an independent, circular loop of DNA.
   - The gene to be transferred (see number 4) is found on the plasmid of the bacterial cell one (see number 3), but not on the plasmid of the bacterial cell two (see number 2).
   - For transfer to occur, a restriction enzyme (see number 5) is needed to remove the gene from the plasmid of the bacterial cell one (see number 2).

- The restriction enzyme works by binding to a specific site on the DNA, cutting it, and releasing the gene to be transferred. After a cell dies and disintegrates, genes are naturally removed and released into the environment.

2. **Step II:**
- Bacterial cell two takes up the gene.
- Note: The integration of genetic material from the environment, considered to be an evolutionary tool, is a common practice among bacterial cells.

3. **Step III:**
- An enzyme, DNA ligase (see number 6), adds the gene to the plasmid of bacterial cell two. The enzyme joins them together by forming chemical bonds between the two segments.

4. **Step IV:**
- The plasmid of bacterial cell two now contains the gene from bacterial cell one (see number 7). Transformation is now complete, with the gene having been transferred from one bacterial cell to another bacterial cell.

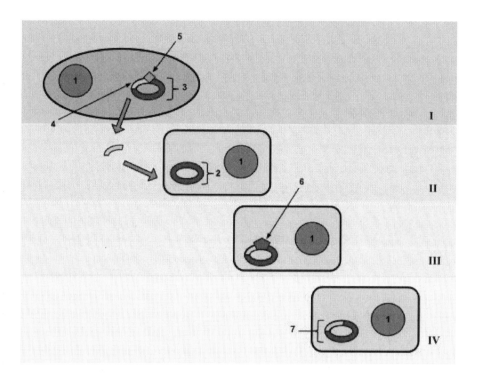

Schematic of bacterial transformation — for which artificial competence must first be induced.

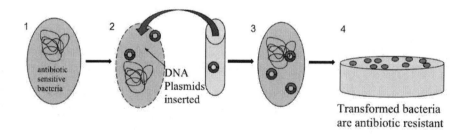

Transformed bacteria are antibiotic resistant

2. Conjugation

Conjugation is the transfer of genetic information with the assistance of **conjugative plasmid.** Unlike transformation, conjugation requires cell-to-cell contact. This exchange of genetic information, which can occur between unrelated bacteria, constitutes a main mechanism of antibiotic resistance transfer.

Conjugation necessitates the presence of a **self-transmissible plasmid** (called an **F plasmid**) in one bacterium. Bacteria that carry F plasmids are referred to as **F (+) cells.** These F plasmids encode the proteins and enzymes necessary for conjugation. During conjugation, a F (+) cell donates (transfers) its F plasmid to a F (-) cell, which in turn makes the recipient cell F (+).

Bacterial conjugation, as illustrated by the schematic diagram below, occurs as follows:

1. **Stage 1:** The donor cell produces pilus – pilus, plural: pili, (sometimes also called fimbria) are hair-like appendages that are found on the surface of many bacterial species.
2. **Stage 2:** Pilus attaches to the recipient cell, drawing both cells together.
3. **Stage 3:** The mobile plasmid is 'nicked' and the single strand of DNA is now transferred to the recipient cell.
4. **Stage 4:** Both cells make another, complementary strand, thus producing a double stranded circular plasmid, all whilst reproducing pili. Both cells are now a viable donor of F-factor (also called fertility factor).

F-plasmid is an **episome** – a genetic element contained in some bacterial cells that allows them to replicate independently of the host. An F-plasmid, which is around 100 kb in length, carries its own origin of replication (or **OriV**) as well as an origin of transfer (or **oriT**). Within each given bacterium, there can only be one copy of F-plasmid, either free or integrated – and a bacterium that possesses such a copy is said to be F-positive or F-plus. The F stands for fertility and cells that luck such (i.e. cells that do not have F-plasmids) are said to be F-negative or F-minus. F-negative or F-minus cells are not capable of conjugation with other bacteria and can only function as recipient cells.

In summary therefore, during conjugation, a F-positive o F-plus bacterium transfers a copy of DNA containing the F-factor to a F-negative bacterium. This transfer makes the previously F-negative or F-minus bacterium capable of producing pilus, rendering it capable of conjugation with other bacteria.

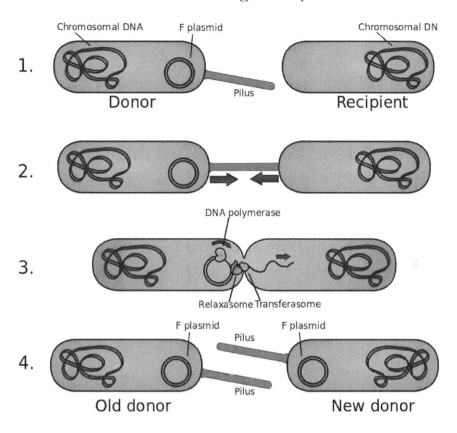

3. Transduction

Transduction, another way by which genetic fragments can be transferred between bacteria, is the process during which a virus infects one bacterial cell and transfers genes (pieces of bacterial DNA) from the infected bacterium to another bacterial cell. Viruses that infect bacteria are called **bacteriophage** or **phage**. Transformation, which is DNAase resistant, does not require physical contact between the 'donor' cell (the cell donating the DNA) and the receiving cell.

There are two types of bacteriophages: virulent phages and temperate phages, and generally speaking, there are also two types of transduction by phage: generalized transduction and specialized transduction.

Generalized transduction: This occurs when the bacteriophage packages any genes – whether chromosomal, plasmid or viral – in a bacterial cell.

Below is a diagram of a typical tailed bacteriophage:

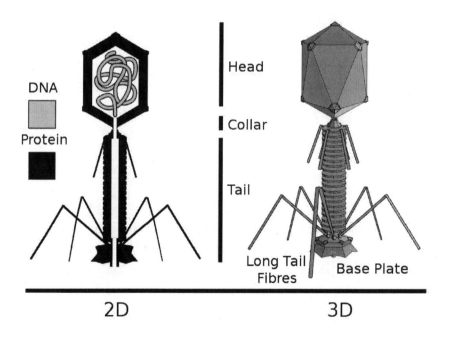

Generalized transduction occurs as follows:

1. Adsorption and penetration – bacterial circular DNA is drawn as a thick circle and viral DNA is drawn as a thin line. Adsorption (the adhesion of a thin layer of molecules or dissolved solids to a surface in a condensed layer) and penetration occur.
    Once the phage has penetrated into a 'host' bacterium, its DNA is transcribed, replicated and translated into enzymes and capsids.
2. Destruction and replication – at the same time (during which transcription, replication and translation occur), bacterial DNA is repressed and destroyed. Destruction of the bacterial DNA leaves some of the thick pieces intact. If these pieces are the same size as the phage DNA, then they may end up being accidentally packed into the phage capsid head. The phage DNA undergoes replication.
3. Translation and packaging – the capsids are translated and packed.
4. Lysis and release of the phages – cell lysis occurs, which liberates the phages (including the phage that contains the bacterial DNA). Following lysis, the phage with the bacterial DNA can go on and infect another bacterium, injecting the bacterial DNA that it is carrying. This newly inserted piece of bacterial DNA may be incorporated if there is some homology between it and the recipient bacterial genome.

Specialized transduction: Whilst generalized transduction is random, specialized transduction occurs when specific DNA fragments (i.e. a restricted set of bacterial genes) are packaged into the bacteriophage, e.g. specific toxin genes or other virulence factors.

Specialized transduction occurs as follows:

1. Specialized transduction occurs with temperate phages, with **phage lambda** in *Escherichia coli*. The temperate phage penetrates and upon penetration, its DNA is incorporated into the bacterial chromosome. At this point, it is called a **prophage** (the genetic material of a phage incorporated into the genome of a bacterium) and the bacterium is said to be **lysogenic** (harboring a temperate *virus* as a prophage or a plasmid). The insertion site of the **lambda prophage** lies between the *Escherichia coli* gene for biotin synthesis and galactose synthesis.

2. Typically, the prophage DNA remains inactive, but it can eventually become active. Once activated, the prophage DNA is spliced out of the bacterial chromosome and is then **replicated translated, and packaged into a capsid**.

3. Sometimes there is an error in splicing and a DNA fragment that lies at one side of the prophage is cut, replicated and packaged with the phage DNA. If such a splicing error occurs, either the biotin gene or the galactose gene is carried with the phage DNA and packaged. This can result in the transfer of a bacterial DNA from one bacterium to another bacterium.

In this way, a bacterium can acquire the gene for galactose synthesis for example (or biotin synthesis) – which it did not previously possess. This type of **gene acquisition** is referred to as **lysogenic conversion.**

Transduction is particularly important as it explains one mechanism through which antibiotic-resistance genes are transferred between bacteria, which in turn leads to the ineffectiveness of antibiotic medications.

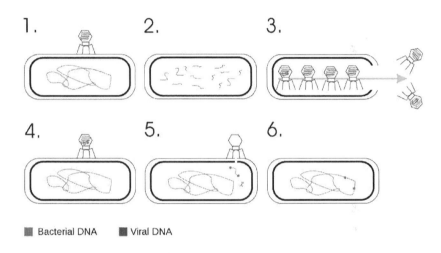

Bacterial DNA   Viral DNA

4. Transposon / Transposition

Transposition occurs when one small DNA piece – called a **transposon** – moves from one location to another location within the DNA of an organism. Transposons, which can carry genes for antibiotic resistance and virulence factors, can insert themselves into a donor chromosome without having DNA homology. Transposons do not replicate independently but instead are copied during the DNA transcription of their host. Transposition necessitates the presence of an enzyme able of cutting and resealing DNA and recognition sites (the site where the enzyme acts). Transposons can be simple or complex, but all lead to DNA modifications.

8. BACTERIAL BINARY FISSION

Most bacteria use binary fission for propagation. Binary fission – the primary method of reproduction of prokaryotic organisms – is a type of asexual cell division, similar to mitosis, during which an organism duplicates its genetic material, dividing into two parts (cytokinesis), with each new organism receiving one copy of DNA, along with the right amount of proteins and nutrients, and everything required for it to function as an independent cell.

Binary fission   Mitosis   Meiosis

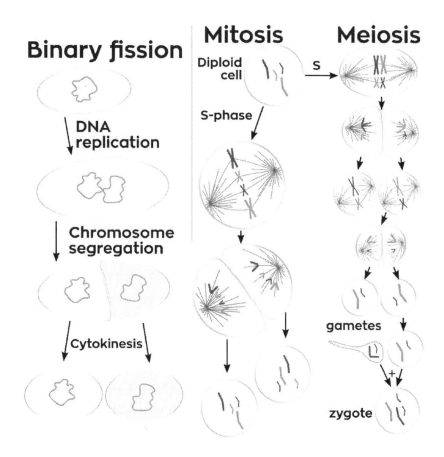

Section 4: Virology – All About Viruses

It is estimated that there are ten times the amount of viral particles than bacterial cells on earth. The diversity of viruses is huge! There are a number of distinctive characteristics that viruses have:

- Viruses have no energy - they drift around until they make contact with a suitable cell.
- They are made up of a **capsid,** which is a protein shell. This encloses the genetic material of the virus.
- Viruses do not have ribosomes or organelles.
- Some viruses have an extra external lipid bilayer membrane. This can contain glycoproteins.
- Certain viruses also include some structural proteins and enzymes within their capsid.
- The genetic material of a virus is either **DNA** or **RNA** – it is never both. The genetic material provides instructions to create millions of clones of the initial virus.
- This reproduction of the genetic material takes place when the virus starts to control the synthetic machinery of the host cell.

In this section we will be exploring the viral structure, viral function, bacteriophage reproduction, virus families, eukaryotes, plant viruses, and host cell defense mechanisms.

1. The Viral Structure

Viruses are made up of **nucleic acid** (the viral genome – either

DNA or RNA) inside of the virus, the **capsid**, and the **envelope**.

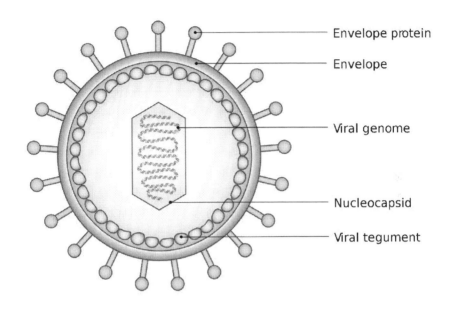

Nucleic Acid

Viruses are either RNA or DNA, and the strands of the nucleic acid can be either single stranded (ss), double stranded (ds).

RNA Viruses

RNA viruses can be either positive stranded (+) or negative stranded (-). When a positive RNA virus arrives at a host cell, its RNA can immediately be translated into protein by the host's ribosomes. Thus, the RNA functions like a messenger RNA (mRNA). In order for negative stranded (-) RNA to be translated, they must first be transcribed into a positive strand (+). This transcription is made by the *RNA-dependent RNA Polymerase,* which is carried in the capsid of the negative stranded (-) RNA.

Notable RNA viruses include: **Retroviruses** (including HIV) possess a unique ability to incorporate into the genome of the host cell. **Reoviridae viruses** (including rotavirus) are the only viruses that have a double stranded (ds) RNA genome.

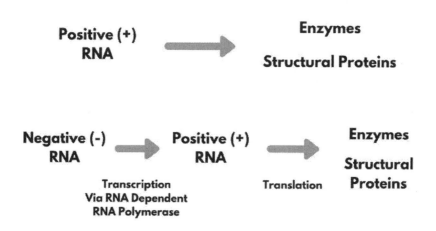

DNA Viruses

DNA viruses are unable to be directly translated into proteins. They must firstly be transcribed into messenger RNA (mRNA). The mRNA can then be translated into structural proteins and enzymes. The majority of DNA viruses have both a positive (+) and negative (-) strand, however only the negative (-) strand of the DNA is read. The positive strand (+) is ignored.

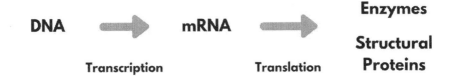

DNA → **mRNA** → **Enzymes**

Structural

Transcription   Translation   **Proteins**

Capsids

The capsid of a virus packages the nucleic acids, allowing it to be delivered to a new host cell. Think of the capsid as structure that provides 'housing' for the genome. When observed microscopically, the capsid of a virus has a geometric appearance, which is the result of symmetrical pattern that is formed by a repeated singular protein or a small number or proteins. There are two types of capsids: *helical* and *icosahedral*.

Helical - The RNA molecule within a helical virus is coated with a protein. The capsid forms a constant helix.

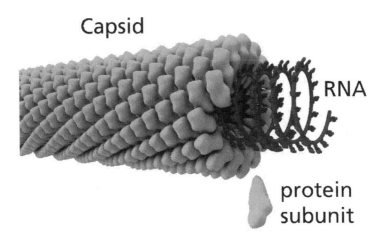

Capsid

RNA

protein
subunit

Icosahedral – A 20-sided shape (icosahedral) makes up the capsid. This creates a spherical shape with the fewest number of proteins possible.

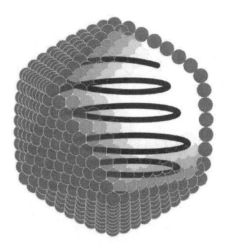

The Envelope

Some viruses have an outer lipid bilayer, an envelope, which surrounds the nucleocapsid. In order to allow the virus to interact with the target cell, the membrane is studded with proteins – often referred to as 'spikes'. The influenza virus, for example, has an envelope comprised of a glycoprotein *hemagglutinin*, and spikes of protein *neuraminidase*. During the final stage of viral replication, the lipid membrane of the host cell is used to create an envelope made up of lipids. Not all viruses have an envelope - such viruses are referred to as *non-enveloped* or *naked viruses*.

Bacteriophage

There are more complex viral structures, such as bacteriophage that infect bacteria. An example of a bacteriophage is shown below.

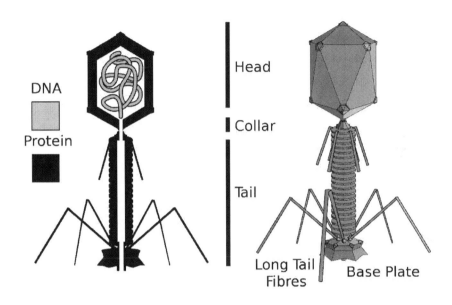

This bacteriophage has an icosahedral head that is joined to a tail via a collar. The tail is equipped with long tail fibres - this structure allows the virus to penetrate the cell wall of bacteria, and then inject viral genetic material within the cell.

2. The Viral Function

Now that we have established the structure of viruses, let's explore how they function to take control of the host cell's machinery to replicate and generate more viral particles. This process is called *viral replication*. The following is the step-by-step process that occurs during viral replication. It is important to note that this process varies between different viral groups.

1. The viral particle becomes attached to the surface of the host cell.

The proteins on the surface of the viral particle interact with the host cell's surface receptors. Thus, this attachment can only happen with host cells that have receptors on their surface. Different host cells have different types of receptors, and therefore the viral attachment is specific for a particular type of cell.

2. The entire virus or the nucleic acid of the virus move inside the host cell.

In order for the transcription to take place, the viral genome must enter the host cell. Any required enzymes for transcription (e.g. reverse transcriptase) must also enter the host cell. The virus then releases its genetic material into the cell – this process is called *uncoating,* and it can happen in a number of ways for different types of viruses:

HIV – An enveloped virus. The envelope is required to access animal cells. The envelope interacts with the cell membrane of the host cell, and then the capsid from the virus moves within the cell.

Influenza – Attaches to the surface of an animal cell, and enters via *endocytosis.*

Advenovirus – An unenveloped virus that enters the host cell via endocytosis.

Bacteriophage – A more complex virus that injects its viral genome into the host cell. The following diagram illustrates the bacteriophage uncoating process.

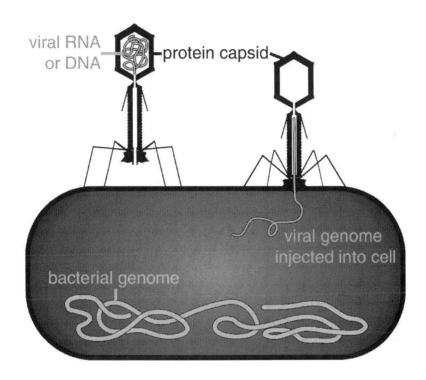

3. The viral genes are transcribed and translated by the host cell.

Initially, viral proteins are created to copy the viral genome and transcribe viral genes. Following this, viral genes are created in large quantities to reproduce the capsid and other parts of the viral structure.

4. The viral proteins are built and the genetic material is placed inside the capsid.

5. Virions (complete viral particles) are discharged from the host cell.

Some of the viral particles take a part of the host cell's membrane, which then becomes their envelope. This process can sometimes cause the cell membrane of the host to *lyse* – the destruction of the cell membrane, which releases its contents.

3.   The Cycles of Viral Reproduction for Bacteriophage

Lytic Phage

The lytic cycle results in a complete destruction of the host's bacterial cell and its membrane. This is called *lysis*. A prime example of this is the much-studied *T4 phage*, which infects the bacterial species *E.Coli*. During the initial stages of T4 infection, the T4 phage creates a large number of virally encoded proteins for the replication of DNA. Thus, there are many copies of the genome within the host cell during the early stage of the infection. Once the capsid and the head have been created they are packaged with DNA, and the tail and fibres are added. By threading a strand of DNA into the genome, the viral genome is added to the head of the phage. Due to the size of the head of the phage, and because the phage copies its genome continuously as a long string, there is always more than one copy of the genome within the virion.

T4 lysozyme is created once all of the viral particles have been assembled. This breaks down the host cell's bacterial wall, which allows the escape of the viral particles, and leaves the host cell in a damaged state. An illustration of the lytic cycle is shown below.

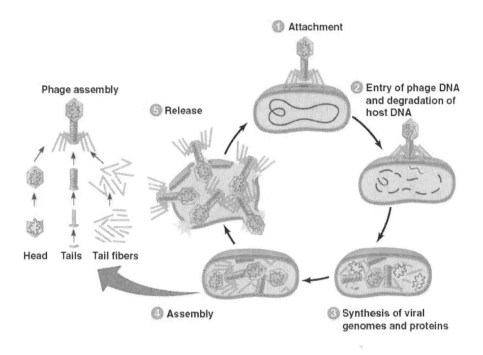

Temperate Phage

A phage can also be temperate, which means it can be either lytic or lysogenic inside the host cell. *Lysogeny* is an approach that viruses can take to promote survival, which allows them to lay dormant for a period of time, instead of continuously searching for new host cells.

A viral genome infects the host cell as a latent prophage, in which there is no initial creation of viral particles. Just one viral protein exists which represses the expression of other viral proteins. At this stage, the bacterial host that contains the prophage is referred to as a *lysogen*. The lysogen can remain in this state throughout a number of generations of bacterial cell divisions. Following this, the prophage can be inducted into a lytic cycle where the viral particles are brought within the host DNA, and viral particles can then be produced. The end result of lysis still occurs similar to that of a lytic phage. Some prophage remain within the DNA of the host and are never inducted into a lytic cycle – these prophage are referred to as a *cryptic viruses*.

An illustration of the lysogenic cycle to the lytic cycle is shown below.

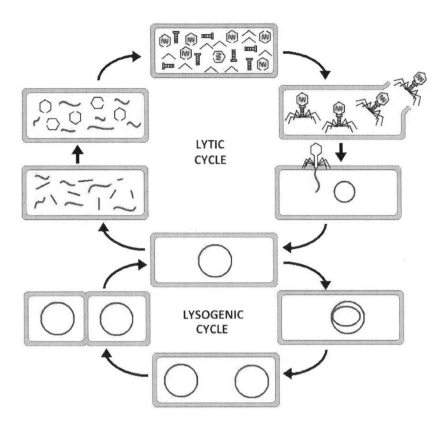

LYTIC
CYCLE

LYSOGENIC
CYCLE

Transposable Phage

Transposable phage not only integrates its genome into the host cell to create a lysogenic cycle, but it also repeats the process as a method for duplicating its genome to induce a lytic cycle. A prime example of transposable phage is *Mu*. When Mu infects bacterial cells, an enzyme named *transposase* rapidly integrates it into the host cell. The transposase makes slices into both strands of the host DNA, and the genome of Mu is placed within the host sequence. This process creates two copies of host sequence on each side of the Mu genome.

If a Mu repressor exists, there will not be an increase in the number of genome copies and there will be no lysing. However, if there is no Mu repressor the transposase enzyme will duplicate the Mu genome to numerous locations. This duplication of a *transposable element* (a movable sequence of DNA) can happen up to 100 times within the genome! *Replicative transposition* refers to when transposable element makes duplicates of themselves, which then move to new locations within the genome. *Conservative transposition* refers to when a sequence of DNA moves to a new location as a complete unit.

4. The Virus Families

We will now summarize the different families of viruses, along with the characteristics that separate them.

DNA Viruses

The majority of DNA viruses are double-stranded and icosahedral, with their replication happening in the nucleus. DNA viruses include:

Herpes (enveloped), **Hepadna** (enveloped), **Adeno** (naked), **Papova** (naked), **Parvo** (naked), **Pox** (enveloped).

There are a couple of DNA viruses that are an exception to the general rules: **Parvovirdae** - only has a single strand.

Poxviridae - although it is double-stranded, it has a complex nature and does not have an icosahedral structure.

RNA Viruses

The general rules of RNA viruses are mostly the opposite to that of DNA viruses. Most RNA viruses are single-stranded (half positive and the other half negative), enveloped, and helical. They generally replicate within the cytoplasm. RNA viruses include:

Corona, Retro, Toga, Picorna, Calici, Reo, Flavi, Paramyxo, Orthomyxo, Bunya, Rhabdo, Arena, Filo.

There are few exceptions to the general rules:

- **Picorna, Calici,** and **Reoviridae** are nonenveloped.
- **Picorna, Reo, Toga, Flavi,** and **Calici** have icosahedral symmetry.
- **Reoviridae** are double stranded.
- **Retro** and **Orthomyxo** replicate in the nucleus.

5. Exploring Eukaryotes

Prokaryotes are viruses that infect bacteria, and *eukaryotes* are viruses that infect animals and plants. There are two key differences between them:

- In the case of bacteria, only the viral genome enters the host cell, whilst the viral particle stays outside. However, for animal viruses the complete virion enters the host cell.

- There is a nucleus within eukaryotes, and viral genes must enter this in order to replicate.

Animal Viruses

Animal viruses are viruses that infect animal cells, and are thus the viruses that make humans unwell. There are animal viruses with each of the different genome types (i.e. single and double stranded DNA and RNA). Most animal viruses are enveloped but some are unenveloped (naked). There are a number of specific properties of animal viruses that are important to know:

- They are viruses that lyse the host cell – they are **virulent**.
- They engage in continuous shedding from the host cell – they are **persistent**.
- They can cause infections that do not cause any consistent disease symptoms – they are **latent**.
- Some animal viruses can cause the fusion of cells – they are **fusogenic**.
- Some animal viruses can cause cancers as a result of generating mutations in the host cell, or manipulation of the regulation of cell growth control.

Animal Virus Example 1: Retroviruses

Retroviruses carry reverse transcriptase, which is a specialized enzyme that duplicates the RNA viral genome into double stranded DNA. Some recognized retroviruses are HIV and a virus called feline leukemia virus (FeLV), which infects cats.

Below is an illustration of the replication cycle of a retrovirus:

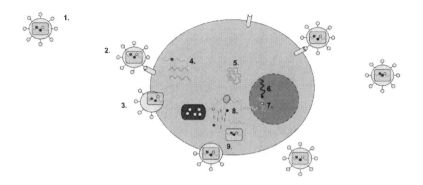

A protein capsid creates the envelope for the retrovirus, which contains two copies of its viral RNA genome. It also contains three viral enzymes that are necessary for infection. There are studded proteins on the envelope, which allows the virus to attach to cells (T-lymphocytes) within the human immune system. Following this, the viral envelope becomes fused with the cell membrane, and the uncoating process of the virus begins. This releases nucleocapsid inside the cytoplasm. The specialized reverse transcriptase then duplicates the RNA genome into double stranded DNA. This enters the nucleus of the host cell and is integrated into the host genome.

Retroviruses such as the HIV virus cannot be removed from the host genome once they have been integrated and become a *provirus* – they do not create an enzyme for excision.

Animal Virus Example 1: Prions

Prions do not have all of the characteristics of a virus, but they are classified as an infectious agent. A prion does not have nucleic acids, but they can infect a neuron, produce the death of cells, and they can be transported from one cell to another. Prions make other proteins non-functional by changing their structure, and this makes the proteins unusable which leads to cell death. Prions only affect animals. If this occurs in the brain of an animal, when prions affect enough neurons it will lead to pain and death. There are a number of forms of prions that affect different types of species:

- Scrapie – affects sheep.
- Bovine spongiform encephalopathy (BSE)/mad cow disease.
- Creuztfeldt-Jakob disease – affects humans.
- Chronic wasting disease – affects deer.

It was once conceived that prions can only be passed between individuals within the same species, but the mad cow prion has been shown to move from cow to human, producing the Creuztfeldt-Jakob disease. Prion proteins target a protein that is typically expressed in all neuronal cells – this is called prion protein (PrP). The normal and prion protein have an identical protein sequence, but are folded in a different manner.

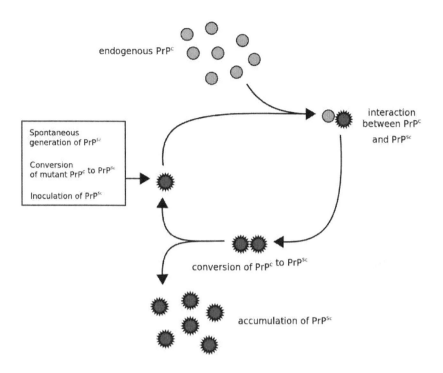

Labeled PrPC ('C' for cellular) is the normal protein with a correct formation. Labeled PrPSc ('Sc' for scrapie, the first prion disease) is the prion protein. PrPSc changes PrPC to PrPSc as it enters the neuron, and this cycle continues as the converted PrPSc convert others to the disease. This creates *amyloids*, which are tightly packed clumps of misfolded proteins.

6. Plant Viruses

Plants can be infected by viruses, including pathogens that affect crops, and *viroids* which are infectious misfolded proteins. The majority of plant viruses are single stranded RNA.

Tobacco Mosaic Virus (TMV)

TMV was the first virus discovered and out of all the plant viruses it is the most studied. It is RNA with a helical structure, comprised of single strand RNA, and encircled by coat proteins.

coiled RNA

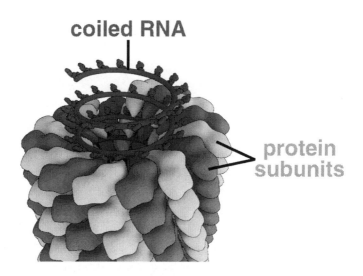

protein
subunits

The genome of the viral RNA is positive, which means that it is the same template for translation that the host cell would use. The uncoating of the viral genome is the first step in the infection. The genome is used for protein translation because it resembles a host mRNA. RNA-dependent RNA polymerase is used to produce a negative RNA duplicate (-RNA) of the genome. Further positive RNA genomes can then be produced from this. Following this, the virus is able to infect other plants as a result of movement proteins and coat proteins. This takes place via cell damage from a herbivore or insect. TMV also uses a method of infection through cell-to-cell connections (*plasmodesmata*). These connections are too small for bacteria to move through, but a movement protein that binds to the viral RNA assists it with entering the neighboring cells to start new infections.

Viroids

Viriods are short RNA sequences that do not have capsid proteins. Viroids enter plant cells following the damage of the cell wall, and via plasmodesmata they are able to move between cells. Although the exact way that viroids cause disease is undetermined, it is predicted that they produce small interfering RNA molecules (siRNA) that affects normal mRNA translation.

7. The Host Cell's Defense Mechanisms

Although the rate of mutation is faster in viruses than in host cells (due to their small genomes), host cells have complex mechanisms to counteract viral replication.

Restriction Enzymes

Bacteria and archaea use enzymes called *restriction enzymes* to break up foreign double stranded DNA that is discovered within the cell. This defense mechanism aims to stop the initiation of the infection cycle – it works to stop bacteriophage genomes that have been introduced into the host cell. Restriction enzymes identify a *recognition sequence* and then proceed to cut double stranded

DNA. This process is referred to as the restriction system. The enzymes are specifically called *restriction endonucleases* because they cut into DNA molecules. The following are some of the particular features of recognition sequences to be aware of:

- Their size is generally 4 to 8 bases.
- They are more likely to occur in a DNA molecule when they have a shorter sequence.
- Their sequence is usually the same in both the forward and reverse direction (*palindromes*).
- Recognition sequences occur in the DNA of all organisms.
- They protect the host cell by preventing the restriction enzyme from binding to the host DNA.
- There are thousands of types of restriction enzymes.

Viruses act against bacterial restriction enzymes by altering their DNA – these processes are called *methylation* and *glucosylation*. Bacteriophages can generate their own restriction enzymes that are then directed at the host DNA. This effectively diminishes any defenses from the host cell.

CRISPR (*Clustered Regularly Interspaced Short Palindromic Repeats*)

There is another mechanism that allows bacteria and archae to not only resist double stranded DNA viruses, but also single stranded DNA/RNA viruses. Within the bacterial genome, short viral sequences recognize and destruct similar viral sequences that appear in the host cell. Although this system is prevalent in bacteria and archaea, its exact workings are not entirely understood.

Illustrated below is an overview of the CRISPR process:

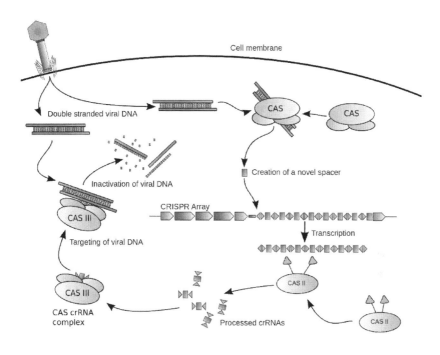

Eukaryotic Defense of RNA Viruses: RNAi

Although eukaryotes do not have a CRISPR mechanism, they can use short RNA sequences the instruct enzymes to break up viral RNA molecules in the cell. There is a system called RNA interference (RNAi) that attends to any recognized double stranded RNA within the cytoplasm. Double stranded RNA viruses only have cells that are double or single stranded RNA. An enzyme called *dicer* cuts up a double stranded RNA molecule that is detected in the cell. It is cut into sections of approximately 21 – 23 base pairs (bp). These sections are called *short interfering RNA* (siRNA) and they are surrounded by RNA-induced silencing complex (RISC). The two RNA strands are split by RISC, and each one aims to discover other single stranded RNA molecules within the cell. These are potentially mRNA being produced by the machinery of the host cell. An enzyme named *slicer* cleaves the single stranded RNA molecules, which stops viral replication.

A visual representation of this process is shown below:

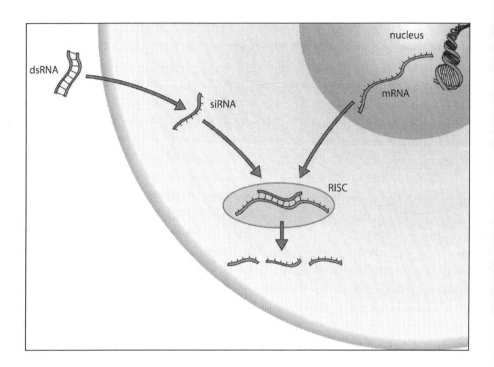

Viruses act to counter this mechanism by creating false RNA's, which then exhaust the Dicer/RISC. They can also avoid RNAi by replicating in areas of the cell that it cannot reach. Finally, viruses can generate proteins that hinder the functioning of the dicer enzyme.

Section 5: Parasitology – All About Parasites

The study of parasites that affect animals and humans is called *parasitology*. Parasites are eukaryotic, and they include *protists* and *worms*.

1. Protists (Protozoa)

Protists are a group of eukaryotic microorganisms containing *phyla*, and they make up the majority of variations within the *Domain Eukarya*. This group is made up of numerous sizes, shapes, and lifestyles. Although most protists are organisms that are single-celled, some form structures that are multicellular (e.g. algae), and some assemble as single cells to form multicellular structures (e.g. some slime molds). The reproduction of protists can involve simple division, or it can involve sophisticated cycles with multiple structures.

We will now explore some examples of protists.

Human Protists

Apicoplexans

Apicoplexans are a group of human parasites that cause very unpleasant (sometimes deadly) diseases. These parasites are unable to live outside of a host, and examples of specific parasites within this group are *Plasmodium*, *Toxoplasma*, and *Cryptosporidium*. A species of plasmodium causes the malaria disease, it has a host within insects and a host within humans. The sexual reproduction of the parasite occurs within the insect (mosquito), and when the mosquito bites a human it transmits motile sporozoites. Within the human, this leads to symptoms of fever and chills, as a result of the asexual reproduction that occurs in the liver and blood. This cycle then continues when a non-infected mosquito bites a human with the disease, and then passes it on to another human. This life cycle is illustrated below:

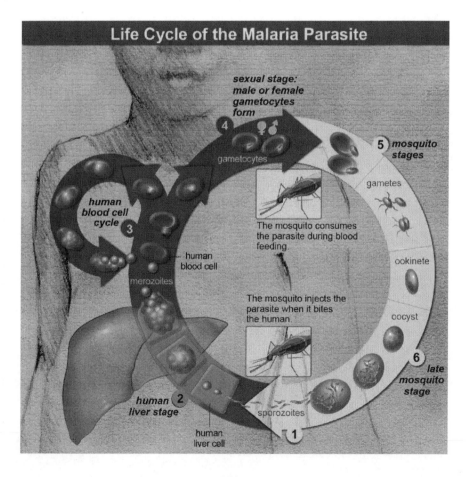

A process called *encystment* allows for the transportation of Cryptosporidium and Toxoplasma between hosts. A cyst containing the organism is created within the host that is then excreted, allowing it to be picked up by other animals. It can then create a new infection by dividing asexually.

Trypanosoma

A disease called African sleeping sickness is caused by a species of Trypanosoma, whereby the parasite enter both the spinal cord and the brain of a human. Similar to malaria, it is spread through a biting insect called the tsetse fly.

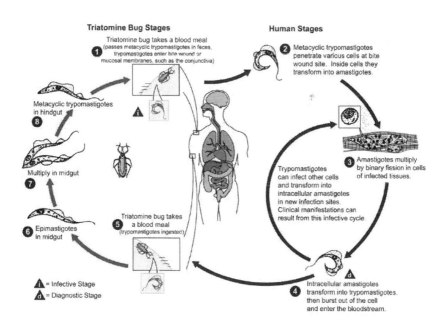

Trypanosoma have a cell shape that is long and slim, and due to its long flagellum beneath its cytoplasmic membrane, it twists when it swims. This allows it to travel in liquids such as blood.

Giardia Lamblia

Giardia lamblia is another parasite with a flagellum that causes a giardiasis, which is a diarrheal disease. It inhabits rivers and streams.

Giardiasis

(Giardia intestinalis)

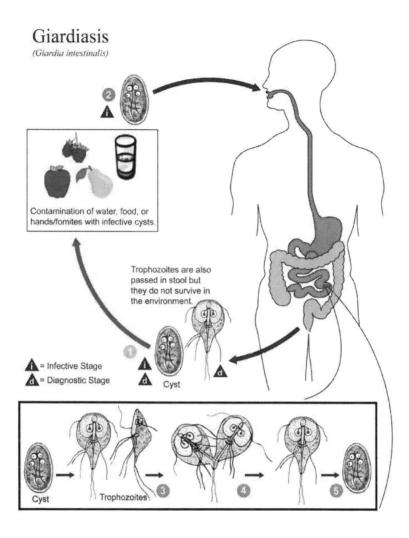

Contamination of water, food, or hands/fomites with infective cysts

Trophozoites are also passed in stool but they do not survive in the environment.

= Infective Stage

= Diagnostic Stage

Cyst

Cyst   Trophozoites

Trichomonas Vaginalis

Trichomonas Vaginalis is another flagellated parasite that is sexually transmitted, but it can live outside the body for short periods of time.

Trichomoniasis
(Trichomonas vaginalis)

🔺 = Infective Stage
🔺 = Diagnostic Stage

Trichomonas vaginalis

1 Trophozoite in vaginal and prostatic secretions and urine

2 Multiplies by longitudinal binary fission

3 Trophozoite in vagina or orifice of urethra

Plant Protists

Oomycetes

Oomycetes cause a number of plant diseases (along with some animal diseases). They break down organic matter that is decaying on forest floors. Examples of plant pathogens from this group are downey and powdery mildews.

Amoeba and Ciliates

Amoeba and *ciliates* are groups of protozoan that are regularly grouped together because they both pursue and digest their food via *phagocytosis*. Phagocytosis is a process that occurs when the cell forms *vacuole,* which is a pocket that is formed around particles of food. Digestive enzymes are then transferred from the cytoplasm to within the vacuole to break down the food particles. Following this, the vacuole opens to discharge the nutrients into the cellular cytoplasm.

A prime example of this group of protozoa is *Paramecium* (cilate). It has *cilia* that move and direct food into the *oral groove*. This food can then be digested via phagocytosis.

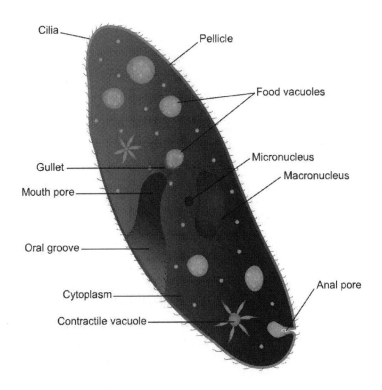

Ciliates are mostly found in environments that are aquatic, either swimming around or feeding whilst attached to surfaces.

Amoeba move around by outwardly extending part of the cell to create a *pseudopodia* - the cytoplasm streams more freely here than in the other parts of the cell. Once the pseudopodia has stretched forward, the contraction of microfilaments pulls forward the other sections of the cell.

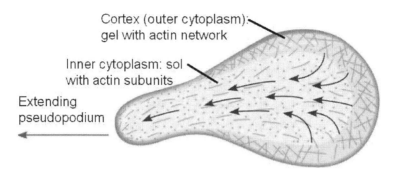

Cortex (outer cytoplasm):
gel with actin network

Inner cytoplasm: sol
with actin subunits

Extending
pseudopodium

Until recently, slime molds were mistaken for fungi due to their production of fruiting bodies throughout reproduction. Despite this, they are now classified to be associated amoeba. Slime molds are either single cell, or they are *plasmodial*, meaning they live as a large mass of protoplasm that contains numerous nuclei and no individual cells. They travel around searching for food in an amoeboid fashion of movement, and they create haploid flagellated cells that form together to produce a new *diploid plasmodium*. Cellular slime molds survive as moving singular haploid cells and when they have consumed all available food they join together to create a slug that becomes stationary. This begins a fruiting process and spores are generated. Each spore subsequently becomes a new singular cell.

Illustrated below is the plasmodial slime mold life cycle:

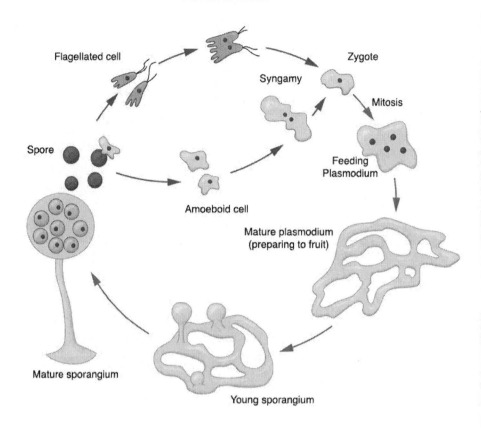

Examining Algae

Algae is a term used to label eukaryotic microorganisms that have chloroplasts within the cell's cytoplasm, and because of this they have a lifestyle that is photosynthetic. A diagram of chloroplast is shown below:

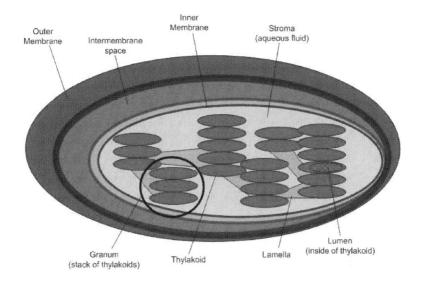

All algae use light energy and release oxygen into their surrounding environment – they are *phototrophs*. They are either single celled or make up simple multicellular structures.

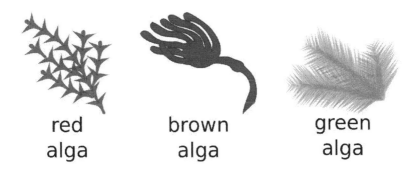

red
alga

brown
alga

green
alga

Algae are generally grouped by their color:

Red algae – its main light-harvesting pigments are *chlorophyll a* and *phycobilisomes*. Their red color is derived from its *phycoerythrin* pigment, which disguises the green color from chlorophyll a. They can either be unicellular or multicellular, and they have the ability to absorb long wavelengths of light in deep water.

Brown algae (*kelp*) - multicellular and can grow rapidly.

Green algae – similar to plants, they contain cellulose within their cell walls, store starch, and use the same chlorophyll. The majority of brown algae are unicellular, but some others are able to create multicellular structures or grow together in a group (*colonial/filamentous*).

Lichen – a combination between single cell green algae and filamentous fungi.

Diatoms – a key component of *photoplankton*. They gain their energy from photosynthesis and accumulate starch as oil. Their cell wall is made up of silica, and the outer part of this is the *frustule* that survives after even after the cell has died.

Radiolarians and Cercozoans – microbes that survive within a structure called *test*, which is made of silica or calium carbonate strengthened organic matter. They feed on bacteria and aquatic matter – they are not photosynthetic. They have thin extendable pseudopodia that collect food.

Dinoflagellates – another key component of oceanic plankton. They have two flagella, allowing them to swim in a spinning motion. Dinoflagellates produce neurotoxins that can have deadly consequences for fish.

2. Helminths (Worms)

Worms are generally macroscopic, and their diagnoses usually involve the visual discovery of eggs within human stool. In this section we will summarize some of the well-known *nematodes* (roundworms) and *platyhelminthes* (flatworms) to give you an understanding of their life cycles. There is generally no immune response to living worms within the normal human host. Despite this, there is usually a marked reaction to dead worms or eggs. The human immune system will elevate *eosinophils* as a response to worm infections, which aids diagnosis.

<u>Nematodes</u>

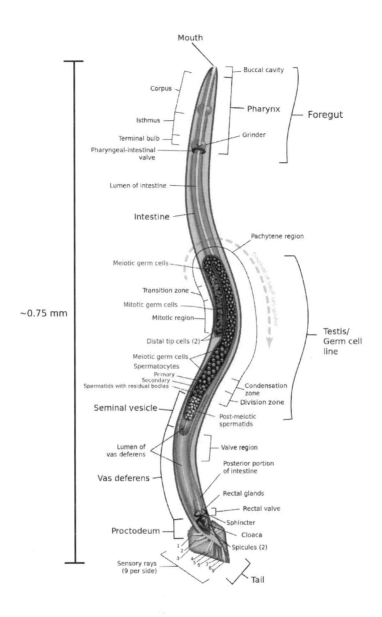

Mouth

Buccal cavity

Corpus

Pharynx

Foregut

Isthmus

Terminal bulb

Grinder

Pharyngeal-intestinal
valve

Lumen of intestine

Intestine

Pachytene region

Meiotic germ cells

Transition zone

Mitotic germ cells

Mitotic region

Testis/
Germ cell
line

Distal tip cells (2)

Meiotic germ cells

Spermatocytes
Primary
Secondary
Spermatids with residual bodies

Condensation
zone

Division zone

Post-meiotic
spermatids

Seminal vesicle

Lumen of
vas deferens

Valve region

Posterior portion
of intestine

Vas deferens

Rectal glands

Rectal valve

Sphincter

Proctodeum

Cloaca

Spicules (2)

Sensory rays
(9 per side)

Tail

~0.75 mm

Intestinal Nematodes

Intestinal nematodes develop into a mature state in the human intestinal tract. In their immature larval forms they can be spread across the body. Different intestinal nematodes are obtained in different ways.

Obtained through the ingestion of eggs: *Ascaris lumbricoides, Trichuris trichiura* (whipworm), and *Enterobius vermicularis* (pinworm).

Obtained through skin (usually foot) penetration of larvae: *Necator americanus* (hookworm) and *Strongyloides stercoralis.*

Obtained through larva in pork meat: *Trichinella spiralis.*

Ascaris lumbricoides, Necator americanus, and Strongyloides stercorous (roundworms) have a larval form, which moves through tissue and then into the lung. They grow in the lung and then are swallowed into the lung, in which they develop into adult worms.

Ascaris lumbricoides: this infection can be minor or show no symptoms at all, but severe cases can involve an adult worm invading the liver, bile ducts, appendix, and gall bladder. The diagnosis is achieved by the discovery of eggs within stool.

Necator americanus and Ancyclostoma duodenale (hookworm): has a comparable lifecycle to ascaris lumbricoides, but their larvae take different routes to reach the lung. Ascaris moves from intestine to lung, but Necator moves from the foot to the lung. Hookworm can cause diarrhea, weight loss, and abdominal pain.

They can also cause an iron deficiency anemia. The diagnosis is achieved by discovering eggs in stool.

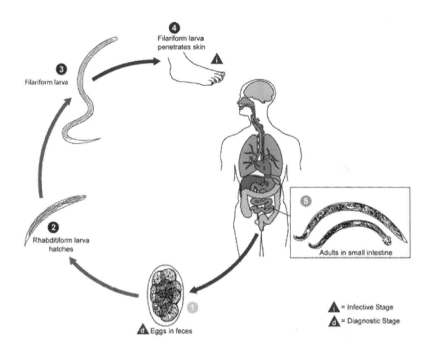

Strongyloides stercoralis: a strongyloide infection can cause abdominal discomfort, vomiting, diarrhea, weight loss, and anemia. The infected patient may also experience lung symptoms and a pruritic rash. Diagnosis is made by discovering larvae in stool.

Trichinella spiralis: infections occur as a result of eating encysted larvae of Trichinella spiralis, frequently found in raw pork. These cysts move to the small intestine and develop into mating adults. The male adult larvae are excreted in feces, but the female larvae move into the intestinal mucosa, and create thousands of larvae. These are then distributed to skeletal muscle and organs via the bloodstream – they can remain here for many years. Many will initially be asymptomatic, but some will experience diarrhea, abdominal discomfort, and fever. Following the invasion of the intestines, the larvae can produce symptoms of muscular aches and fever. The diagnosis is made with biopsy of the muscle and serologic tests, which will uncover encysted larvae.

Trichuris trichiura (whipworm): Trichuris trichiura and Enterobius vermicularis have very basic life cycles with no tissue invasion and no involvement with the lungs. Transmission of Trichuris trichiura takes place through infective eggs that have contaminated food. Once ingested, the eggs hatch and travel to the large intestine. An infected patient may experience pain and diarrhea. Diagnosis is achieved through the discovery of eggs in feces.

Enterobius vermicularis (pinworm) – when the eggs are ingested, the pinworms develop in the cecum and the large intestine. The perianal area becomes infected as a result of the female pinworms, and this causes perianal itching. Diagnosis is achieved using scotch tape on the anal area to capture and find eggs.

The treatment of all intestinal nematodes mentioned above involves the use of the same drugs (*Mebendazole, Thiabendazole, Albendazole*), which paralyze the worms and force them to be excreted in stool. An alternative drug for Enterobius vermicularis (pinworm), Necator americanus (hookworm), and Ascaris lumbricoides is *pyrantel pamoate*.

Blood and Tissue Nematodes

Instead of spreading through fecal contamination, blood and tissue nematodes are spread by the bite of an arthropod. Arthropods are round, threadlike worms called *filariae* that survive in lymphatic tissue and produce *microfilariae*. Microfilariae move through tissue and travel in the bloodstream and lymphatic system. Bloodsucking arthropods extract microfilariae and pass them onto another human. Allergic reactions to microfilariae and dead worms cause disease.

Onchocerca volvulus: infected black flies bite humans to transmit larvae (microfilariae), which produce this filarial infection. The mature larvae are found in subcutaneous tissue fibrous nodules within the skin. More microfilariae are produced as a result of mating, and they move through connective tissue. Those infected will experience a pruritic rash and the skin may become dry and scaly. Larvae can also travel to the eye, which can cause blindness. Diagnosis is usually made from the discovery of microfilariae in skin biopsies. Onchocerciasis can be treated using a new drug called ivermectin, which kills the larvae and stops the reproduction of microfilariae.

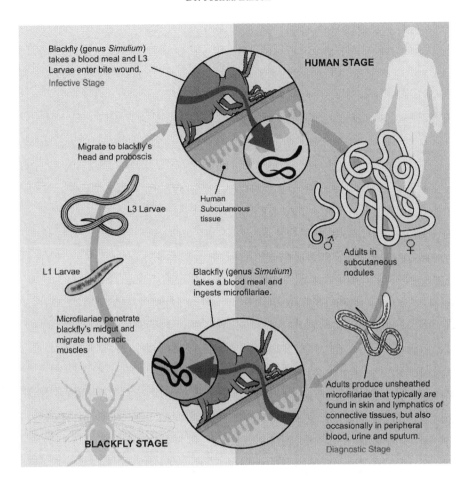

Wuchereria bancroPi and Brugia malayi (Elephantiasis): causes chronic swelling of the leg as a result of a lymphatic infection. The transmission of microfilariae occurs through a bite of an infected mosquito. The microfilariae develop into their mature form within the lymphatic vessels and lymph nodes of the lower extremities and lymph nodes. The offspring of microfilariae from adults migrate to nearby blood vessels. Minor infections will likely only produce enlarged lymph nodes, but more severe infections can result febrile episodes, involving enlarged inguinal lymph nodes and headaches. Continuous exposures will result in fibrous tissue that clusters around dead filariae inside lymph nodes, which creates leg and genital swelling. Diagnosis is generally made by identifying microfilariae within the blood during night hours. Treatment is made using the agent Diethylcarbamazine.

Dracunculus medinensis (Guinea worm): contamination occurs as a result of drinking water that contains microscopic crustaceans, which are larvae that enter the intestine and migrate into subcutaneous tissue. The larvae then grow into adults and mate – the female can grow up to 100cm in length over the period of year. Symptoms of dracunculus medinensis include vomiting, nausea, hives, and breathlessness. Treatment is made by a direct physical removal of the worm.

Section 6: Mycology – All About Fungi

Fungi are eukaryotic cells that cannot produce energy through photosynthesis because they do not have chlorophyll. In this section we will be exploring the different categories of fungi that can cause disease.

Yeast: A growth form of fungi that are unicellular and they appear through budding. They can develop into long forms of yeast cells when the buds do not separate.

Hyphae: Filamentous structures made up of fungal cells.

Molds (Mycelia): Made up of intertwined branching hyphae that form multicellular colonies. They produce spores.

Spores: The reproductive unit of molds.

Dimorphic fungi: Depending on environmental conditions, these fungi are able to grow as yeast or mold. They generally grow as yeast at body temperature.

Saprophytes: Fungi that survive in and feed off organic matter.

The Fungal Structure

The cell membrane: The layer surrounding the fungal cytoplasm. It contains an essential sterol called *ergosterol*. Antifungal agents work to interrupt ergosterol.

The cell wall: The majority of the cell wall is made up of carbohydrate, along with smaller amounts of protein. The fungal cell wall is an antigen to the immune system of humans.

The capsule: A coating surrounding the cell wall that is made up of polysaccharides.

Superficial Fungal Infections

Superficial fungal infections do not cause any symptoms, apart from a pigment change in the skin.

Pityriasis versicolor (tinea versicolor): Causes hypopigmented or hyperpigmented skin patches. It is caused by Malassezia fur fur.

Tinea nigra: Causes dark brown/black skin patches on the soles of the feet and hands. The patches occur due to a harmless infection by Exophiala werneckii.

Diagnosis of superficial fungal infections is achieved by microscopic examination of scrapings from the skin, combined with potassium hydroxide (KOH). As the potassium hydroxide digests any debris that is nonfungal, hyphae and spherical yeast will be revealed. The treatment generally involves applying selenium sulfide anti-dundruff shampoo.

Cutaneous Fungal Infections: Skin, Hair, and Nails

Dermatophytoses

A group of cutaneous fungal infections, which are initiated by over 30 species of fungi. Dermatophytic fungi survive in the dead layers (see stratum corneum layer below) of skin, hair, and nails. They produce *kerarinase*, which is an enzyme that digests keratin. This results in the skin becoming scaly, hair loss, and nail crumbling. *Microsporum, Trichophyton,* and *Epidermophyton* are common dermatophytes.

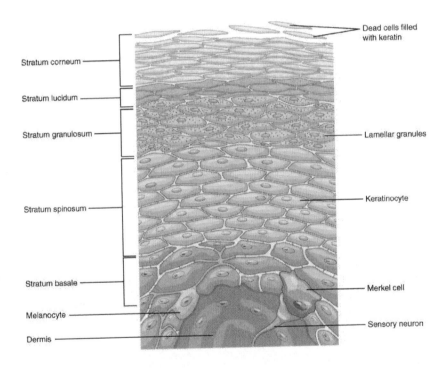

Tinea corporis (also called 'ringworm'): After an outbreak in the stratum corneum, the fungi cause a red shaped ring on the surface of the skin.

Tinea cruris ('jock itch'): Causes itchy red patches around the groin area and the scrotum.

Tinea pedis ('athlete's foot'): Causes the cracking and peeling of skin between the toes. It occurs as a result of moisture and warmth.

Tinea capitis: Fungal organisms develop in the hair and scalp, which results in red scaly lesions and hair loss.

Tinea unguium: Results nails that become thickened, brittle, and discolored.

The diagnosis of a dermatophyte infection generally involves microscopic examination to discover branched hyphae, and directly examining the hair and skin with a Wood's ultraviolet light. The treatment includes the application of topical imidazoles, and oral agents (terbinafine, the azoles) for more severe dermatophyte infections.

Candida Albicans

Candida albicans cause another type of cutaneous fungal infection. Candida can cause oral thrush, diaper rash, and a vaginal infection called candida vaginitis.

Subcutaneous Fungal Infections

Following trauma to the skin, subcutaneous fungal infections can gain entry to the body. They either remain in the subcutaneous tissue, or they migrate to local lymph nodes. These fungi survive in soil and have a low level of virulence.

Sporothrix schenckii (Sporotrichosis): a dimorphic fungi that is often discovered in soil and on plants. A prick from a thorn contaminated with Sporothrix schenckii creates a nodule that becomes necrotic and begins to ulcerate. More nodules are then formed nearby and up the lymphatic tracts. When this fungus is examined microscopically it reveals yeast that reproduces via budding. When the culture is at 37°C it is in a yeast form, and when at 25 °C it is branching hyphae. The treatment involves itraconazole, fluconazole, and oral potassium iodide.

Phialophora and Cladosporium (Chromoblastomycosis): a subcutaneous infection, which is initiated by *Phialophora* and *Cladosporium* – these are soil saprophytes living on rotten wood. The infection occurs as a result of a wound, which then develops into small lesion. Following this, additional violet colored lesions form nearby. Diagnosis is made with the discovery of copper colored sclerotic bodies (with KOH). The treatment involves itraconazole and local excision.

Systemic Fungal Infections

Histoplasma capsulatum, Blastomyces dermatitidis, and *Coccidioides immitis* all cause systemic disease in humans. They are all dimorphic fungi that grow in mycelial forms with spores (at 25 °C on Sabouraud's agar) and in a yeast form (at 37 °C on blood agar). They inhabit soil and release spores into the environment, allowing humans to inhale them and thus they grow as yeast cells at body temperature.

The Mechanism of Disease

All three of the systemic fungal infections have a comparable mechanism of disease, which is similar to that of tuberculosis. Similar to *Mycobacterium tuberculosis*, the three fungi are obtained via inhalation. Despite this, there are two key differences: the fungal infections are acquired in a spore form, and they are not spread between people. The spores get into the environment via vegetation, soil, and bird droppings. Once the spores have been inhaled, a local infection occurs in the lung. Following this, the spores are disseminated in the bloodstream. At this point, the fungi are generally killed by the *cellmediated immune system.*

All three fungi have three distinct clinical features:

- **Asymptomatic** - most cases show no symptoms.
- **Disseminated** – the fungi can cause disseminated disease (although this is rare).
- **Pneumonia** – minor pneumonia can occur, along with a cough and fever. Some rare cases develop severe pneumonia.

The diagnosis of the three fungal infections can involve a biopsy of the tissue affected. Silver stain can be used to examine the tissue for yeast. Serologic tests can also be used, along with a urine histoplasma antigen test. There is usually no treatment needed for acute pulmonary histoplasmosis and coccidioidomycosis. In chronic or disseminated cases, itraconazole/amphotericin B is often necessary for a number of months. Blastomyces cases require amphotericin B/itraconazole treatment.

Dr. Joshua Larsen

Section 7: Final Notes

"We cannot fathom the marvelous complexity of an organic being; but on the hypothesis here advanced this complexity is much increased. Each living creature must be looked at as a microcosm – a little universe, formed of a host of self-propagating organisms, inconceivably minute and as numerous as the stars in heaven."

- *Charles Darwin*

I would like to take this opportunity to thank you for purchasing this book. I hope you have now acquired a good understanding of microbial life and the impact of this invisible world on our everyday lives. Of course, microbiology is an essential science that continues to progress and I do encourage everyone to continue their exploration, as there is always more to discover and learn.

I sincerely wish you the best of luck and the best of health. If you feel you have gained some valuable knowledge from this book, I would really love to hear any feedback that you may have. Reviews can be left on the Amazon book page. I look forward to hearing from you!

Best wishes,
Dr. Joshua Larsen

Made in the USA
San Bernardino, CA
10 June 2019